HATHA YOGA

other recent books on similar topic

ENCYCLOPAEDIA OF TANTRA. in 5 Volumes
Edited by Sadhu Santideva *Bestseller*

ENCYCLOPAEDIA OF BUDDHIST TANTRA. in 5 Volumes
Edited by Sadhu Santideva

ENCYCLOPAEDIA OF INDIAN MYSTICISM. in 12 Volumes
Edited by Sadhu Santideva *Bestseller*

RITUALS AND PRACTICES OF TANTRA. in 3 Volumes
Gaurinath Sastri

THERAPEUTIC TANTRA.
The Power of Physical, Psychological, and Spiritual Healing
Edited by Gaurinath Sastri

INTRODUCTION TO TANTRA. in 2 Volumes
Gaurinath Sastri

Also Available . . .

THE HINDUS.
Encyclopaedia of Hinduism in 5 Volumes
Edited by Subodh Kapoor *Bestseller*

THE BUDDHISTS.
Encyclopaedia of Buddhism in 5 Volumes
Edited by Subodh Kapoor

ENCYCLOPAEDIA OF INDIAN HERITAGE. in 90 Volumes
A Descriptive Work of Indological Research in Philosophy, Religion, Sacred Literature, Society, Thought, Traditions, and Ancient Sciences.
Edited by Subodh Kapoor

HINDU MYSTICISM.
Studies in Vaisnavism and Tantricism in 2 Volumes
By Mahendra Natha Sarkar

Mysticism in Bhagavat Gita.
By Mahendranatha Sircar

HATHA YOGA

OR

THE YOGI PHILOSOPHY OF

PHYSICAL WELL BEING

By

Yogi Ramacharaka

AUTHOR OF "SCINCE OF BREATH", "YOGI PHILOSOPHY AND ORIENTAL OCCULTISM", ETC.

WITH NUMEROUS EXERCISES, ETC.

Cosmo Publications

2004 New Delhi

HATHA YOGA
or the Yogi Philosophy of Well Being

First Published by COSMO 2004

ISBN 81-7755-754-8

Published by
MRS. RANI KAPOOR
for COSMO PUBLICATIONS
Publishing Division of
GENESIS PUBLISHING PVT. LTD.
24-B, Ansari Road, Darya Ganj,
New Delhi-110 002, INDIA

Printed at
Mehra Offset Press

TABLE OF CONTENTS

PUBLISHERS' NOTICE

OUR original intention, when we arranged for the publication of this book, and, in fact, almost up until it went to press, was that it should be, in a measure, supplementary to our little book, " Science of Breath " by the same author—that is to say, it should take up the subject of " Hatha Yoga " with the exception of that phase of the subject (breathing, etc.) which has been covered in that book. But at the last moment we decided that it would be a mistake to publish a book on " Hatha Yoga " with such an important part of the subject as Yogi Breathing omitted, even though that subject had been covered in another book. To omit that important phase of the subject would be working an injustice to those who purchased the new book, as many of such purchasers would never have read the first book, and would be justified in expecting that the present book would treat of all phases of the general subject. So we decided to incorporate in the present volume those parts of " Science of Breath " which belonged strictly to the subject of " Hatha Yoga," omitting such portions as belonged rather to the other branch of the Yogi Philosophy, *i.e.*, Raja Yoga. We mention these facts that the purchasers of this book, who have also read our former book, might not accuse us of filling a new book with parts of an old one. We advertised this book, intending to give only the supplemental parts, as above stated, and the portions of " Science of Breath," which have been added thereto, have been inserted at our own expense, and in the nature of " good measure," or the " baker's dozen."

It is probable that, at some future time, we will make arrangements with the same author to take up the "Raja Yoga" portions of "Science of Breath," and to amplify and enlarge upon same, adding to the foundation already built, just as he has done in the present book upon the "Hatha Yoga" foundation contained in the little book first published by us. If this course is followed, the present book, "HATHA YOGA," will be the first of a series of "Yogi Books," taking up, in succession, the different phases of the great Yogi Philosophy, the little book "Science of Breath" serving as an introduction to the series, and as a handy little book for beginners, or those just becoming interested in the subject.

"HATHA YOGA," the present book, deals altogether with the physical. The psychical, mental and spiritual phases of the subject belong to the other branches of the work. "Hatha Yoga," however, will be a splendid foundation upon which the student may build, as a sound, strong, healthy body is necessary for one to do his best work and study, as the author of this book has so well explained in the text.

We have asked the author to write a preface to this book, but this he declines to do, as he feels that the book should speak for itself, and he does not like the idea of (as he expresses it) "intruding his personality" upon his readers, holding that truth should be self-evident and needing no personal touch to make it truth. This notice, therefore, will take the place of a preface in this case.

YOGI PUBLICATION SOCIETY.

TO THE

HEALTHY MAN AND WOMAN

THIS BOOK

IS RESPECTFULLY DEDICATED.

THEY HAVE DONE CERTAIN THINGS (CONSCIOUSLY OR SUB-CONSCIOUSLY) IN ORDER TO BRING THEMSELVES FROM INFANCY TO HEALTHY, NORMAL MATURITY, AND IF YOU (WHO MAY NOT BE SO HEALTHY AND NORMAL) WILL DO JUST THESE SAME THINGS, THERE IS NO REASON WHY YOU, TOO, SHOULD NOT BE JUST AS ARE THEY. AND THIS LITTLE BOOK IS OUR ATTEMPT TO TELL YOU JUST WHAT THIS HEALTHY MAN AND WOMAN DID IN ORDER TO BE JUST WHAT THEY ARE.

READ IT, AND THEN GO AND DO LIKEWISE, SO FAR AS YOU ARE ABLE.

IF YOU DOUBT THE TRUTH OF OUR STATEMENTS, FIND SOME HEALTHY MAN OR WOMAN, AND WATCH HIM, OR HER, CLOSELY, AND SEE WHETHER HE, OR SHE, DOES NOT DO THE THINGS WE HAVE POINTED OUT TO YOU TO DO IN THIS BOOK—AND WHETHER HE, OR SHE, DOES NOT LEAVE UNDONE THE THINGS WE HAVE ASKED YOU TO AVOID. WE ARE WILLING TO SUBMIT OUR TEACHINGS TO THIS SEVERE

— TEST — APPLY IT. —

CHAPTER I

WHAT IS HATHA YOGA?

THE science of Yoga is divided into several branches. Among the best known and leading divisions are (1) Hatha Yoga; (2) Raja Yoga; (3) Karma Yoga; (4) Gnani Yoga. This book is devoted only to the first named, and we will not attempt to describe the others at this time, although we will have something to say upon all of these great branches of Yoga, in future writings.

Hatha Yoga is that branch of the Yogi Philosophy which deals with the physical body—its care—its well-being—its health—its strength—and all that tends to keep it in its natural and normal state of health. It teaches a natural mode of living and voices the cry which has been taken up by many of the Western world: "Let us get back to Nature," excepting that the Yogi does not have to *get* back, for he is already there, for he has always clung close to nature and her ways, and has not been dazzled and befooled by the mad rush towards externals which has caused the modern civilized races to forget that such a thing as nature existed. Fashions and social ambitions have not reached the Yogi's consciousness—he smiles at these things, and regards them as he does the pretences of childish games—he has not been lured from nature's arms, but continues to cuddle close up to the bosom of his good mother who has always given him nourishment, warmth and protection. Hatha Yoga is first, nature; second, *nature*, and last, NATURE. When confronted with a choice of methods, plans, theories, etc., apply to them the touchstone: "Which is the natural way?" and always choose that which seems to conform the nearest to nature. This plan will be a good one for our students to follow when their attention is directed to the many theories; "fads"; methods; plans and ideas, along health lines, with which the Western world is being flooded. For instance, if they are asked to believe that they are in danger of losing their "magnetism," by coming in contact with the earth, and are advised to wear rubber soles and heels upon their shoes, and to sleep in beds "insulated" with glass feet, to prevent nature (mother Earth) from sucking and drawing out of them the magnetism which she has just given them, let the students ask themselves "What does Nature say about this?" Then, in order to find out what nature says, let them see whether nature's plans could have contemplated the manufacture and wearing of rubber soles, and glass feet for beds Let them see whether the strong magnetic men, full of vitality, do these things—let them see whether the most vigorous races in the world have done these things—let them see whether they feel debilitated from lying down on the grassy sward, or whether the natural impulse of man is not to fling himself upon the grassy bank—let them see whether the natural impulse of childhood is not to run barefoot; whether it does not refresh the feet to take off the shoes (rubber soles and all) and walk around barefooted; whether rubber boots are particularly conducive to "magnetism" and vitality, and so on. We give this merely as an illustration, not that we wish to waste time in discussing the merits or demerits of rubber soles, and glass bed feet as a preservative of magnetism. A little observation will teach the man that all of nature's answers show him that he gets much of his magnetism from the earth, and that the earth is a battery charged with it. and is always willing and anxious to give forth its strength to man, instead of being devoid of it and to be dreaded as being anxious and likely to "draw" the magnetism from man, its child. Some of these latter day prophets will next be teaching that the air draws Prana from people, instead of giving it to them.

So, by all means, apply the nature test to all theories of this kind—our own included—and if they do not square with nature, discard them—the rule is a safe one. Nature knows what it is about—she is your friend and not your enemy.

There have been many and most valuable works written on the other branches of the Yogi Philosophy, but the subject of Hatha Yoga has been dismissed with a brief reference by most of the writers upon Yoga. This is largely due to the fact that in India there exists a horde of ignorant mendicants of the lower fakir class, who pose as Hatha Yogis, but who have not the slightest conception of the underlying principles of that branch of Yoga. These people content themselves with obtaining control over some of the involuntary muscles of the body (a thing possible to anyone who will devote to it the time and trouble necessary for its accomplishment), thereby acquiring the ability to perform certain abnormal " tricks " which they exhibit to amuse and entertain (or disgust) Western travellers. Some of their feats are quite wonderful, when regarded from the standpoint of curiosity, and the performers would be worthy applicants for paying positions in the " dime museums " of America, indeed their feats being very similar to some performed by some of the Western " freaks." We hear of these people exhibiting with pride such tricks and acquired habits as, for instance, the ability to reverse the peristaltic action of the bowels and intestines, and the swallowing movements of the gullet, so as to give a disgusting exhibition of a complete reversal of the normal processes of those parts of the body, so that articles introduced into the colon may be carried upwards and ejected from the gullet, by this reverse movement of the involuntary muscles, etc. This, from a physician's point of view is most interesting, but to the layman is a most disgusting thing, and one utterly unworthy of a man. Other feats of these so-called Hatha Yogis are about on a par with the instance which we have reluctantly given, and we know of nothing that they perform which is of the slightest interest or benefit to the man or woman seeking to maintain a healthy, normal, natural body. These mendicants are akin to the class of fanatics in India who assume the title " Yogi," and who refuse to wash the body for religious reasons ; or who sit with uplifted arm until it is withered ; or who allow their finger nails to grow until they pierce their hands ; or who sit so still that the birds build nests in their hair; or who perform other ridiculous feats, in order to pose as "holy men" before the ignorant multitude, and, incidentally, to be fed by the ignorant classes who consider that they are earning a future reward by the act. These people are either rank frauds, or self-deluded fanatics, and as a class are on a par with a certain class of beggars in American and European large cities who exhibit their self-inflicted wounds, and bogus deformities, in order to wring pennies from the passer-by, who turns his head and drops the coppers in order to get the thing out of his sight.

The people whom we have just mentioned are regarded with pity by the real Yogis who regard Hatha Yoga as an important branch of their philosophy, because it gives man a healthy body—a good instrument with which to work—a fitting temple for the Spirit.

In this little book, we have endeavoured to give in a plain, simple form, the underlying principles of Hatha Yoga—giving the Yogi plan of physical life. And we have tried to give you the reason for each plan. We have found it necessary to first explain to you in the terms of Western physiology the various functions of the body, and then to indicate Nature's plans and methods, which one should adhere to as far as possible. It is not a "doctor book," and contains nothing about medicine, and practically nothing about the cure of diseases, except where we indicate what one should do in order to get back to a natural state. Its keynote is the Healthy Man—its main purpose to help people to conform to the standard of the normal man. But we believe that that which keeps a healthy man healthy will make an unhealthy man healthy, if he follows it. Hatha Yoga preaches a sane, natural, normal manner of living and life, which, if followed, will benefit anyone. It keeps close to nature and advocates a return to natural methods in preference to those which have grown up around us in our artificial habits of living.

This book is simple—very simple—so simple, in fact, that many will most likely throw it aside because it contains nothing new or startling. They have probably hoped for some wonderful recital of the far-famed freak tricks of the mendicant Yogis (?) and plans whereby these feats could be duplicated by those who would read it. We must tell such people that this book is not that kind of book. We do not tell you how to assume seventy-four kinds of postures, nor how to draw linen through the intestines for the purpose of cleaning them out (contrast this with nature's plans), or how to stop the heart's beating, or to perform tricks with your internal apparatus. Not a bit of such teaching will you find here. We *do* tell you how to command a rebellious organ to again function properly, and several other things about the control over an involuntary part which has gone on a strike, but we have mentioned these things only in the line of making man a healthy being—not to make a "freak" of him.

We have not said much about disease. We have preferred to hold up to your gaze the Healthy Man and Woman, asking you to look well at them and see what makes them healthy and keeps them healthy. Then we call your attention to what they do and how they do it. Then we tell you to go and do likewise, if you would be like them. That is all we try to do. But that "all" is about everything that may be done for you—you must do the rest yourself.

In other chapters, we tell you why the Yogis take care of the body, and also the underlying principle of the Hatha Yoga—that belief in the Intelligence behind all Life—that trust in the great Life Principle to carry on its work properly—that belief that if we will but rely on that great principle, and will allow it to work in and through us all will be well with our bodies. Read on, and you will see what we are trying to say to you—will get the message which we have been charged to deliver to you. In answer to the question, with which this chapter is headed: "What is Hatha Yoga?" we say to you: Read this book to the end, and you will understand some little about what it really is—to find out *all* it is put into practice the precepts of this book, and you will get a good fair start on the road to that knowledge you seek.

CHAPTER II

THE YOGIS' REGARD FOR THE PHYSICAL BODY

To the casual observer, the Yogi Philosophy presents the apparent anomaly of a teaching which, while holding that the physical body is material and as nothing when compared to the higher principles of Man, at the same time devotes much care and importance to the instruction of its students in the direction of the careful attention, nourishment, training, exercise and improvement of that physical body. In fact one whole branch of the Yogi teachings, Hatha Yoga, is devoted to this care of the physical body, and goes into considerable detail regarding the instruction of its students in the principles of this physical training and development.

Some Western travellers in the Orient who have seen the care which the Yogis bestow upon their bodies, and the time and attention which they devote to the task, have jumped to the conclusion that the Yogi Philosophy is merely an Oriental form of Physical Culture, a little more carefully studied, perhaps, but a system having nothing "spiritual" in it. So much for seeing merely the outer forms, and not knowing enough to look "behind the scenes."

We scarcely need to explain to our students the real reason for the Yogis' care for the body, nor need we apologize for the publication of this little book which has for its end the instruction of Yogi students in the care and scientific development of the physical body.

The Yogis believe, you *know*, that the *real* Man is not his body. They know that the immortal "I" of which each human being is conscious to a greater or lesser degree, is not the body which it merely occupies and uses. They know that the body is but as a suit of clothes which the Spirit puts on and off from time to time. They know the body for what it is, and are not deceived into the belief that it is the real Man. But while knowing these things, they also know that the body is the instrument in which, and by which the Spirit manifests and works. They know that the fleshly covering is necessary for Man's manifestation and growth in this particular stage of his development. They know that the body is the Temple of the Spirit. And they, consequently, believe that the care and development of the body is as worthy a task as is the development of some of the higher parts of Man, for with an unhealthy and imperfectly developed physical body the mind cannot function properly, nor can the instrument be used to the best advantage by its master, the Spirit.

It is true that the Yogi goes beyond this point, and insists that the body be brought under the perfect control of the mind—that the instrument be finely turned so as to be responsive to the touch of the hand of the master.

But the Yogi knows that the highest degree of responsiveness on the part of the body may be obtained only when it, the body, is properly cared for, nourished and developed. The highly trained body must, first of all, be a strong healthy body. For these reasons the Yogi pays such great attention and care to the physical side of his nature, and, for the same reason, the Oriental system of Physical Culture forms a part of the Yogi science of Hatha Yoga.

The Western Physical Culture enthusiast develops his body for his body's sake, often believing that the body is He. The Yogi develops the body knowing it to be but an instrument for the use of the real part of himself, and solely that he may perfect the instrument to the end that it be used in the work of Soul growth. The Physical Culturist contents himself with mere mechanical movements and exercises for developing the muscles. The Yogi throws Mind into the task, and develops not only the muscle but every organ, cell, and part of his body as well. Not only does he do this, but he obtains control over every part of his body, and acquires mastery over the involuntary part of his organism as well as over the voluntary, something of which the average Physical Culturist knows practically nothing.

We trust to point out to the Western student the way of the Yogi teachings regarding the perfecting of the physical body, and feel assured that he who will follow us carefully and conscientiously will be amply rewarded for his time and trouble, and will acquire the feeling of mastery, over a splendidly developed physical body, of which body he will feel as proud as does the master violinist of the Stradivarius which responds almost with intelligence to the touch of his bow, or as does the master artisan over some perfect tool which enables him to create beautiful and useful things for the world.

CHAPTER III

THE WORK OF THE DIVINE ARCHITECT

THE Yogi Philosophy teaches that God gives to each individual a physical machine adapted to his needs, and also supplies him with the means of keeping it in order, and of repairing it if his negligence allows it to become inefficient. The Yogis recognize the human body as the handiwork of a great Intelligence. They regard its organism as a working machine, the conception and operation of which indicates the greatest wisdom and care. They know that the body IS because of a great Intelligence, and they know that the same Intelligence is still operating through the physical body, and that as the individual falls in with the working of the Divine Law, so will he continue in health and strength. They also know that when Man runs contrary to that law, inharmony and disease result. They believe that it is ridiculous to suppose that this great Intelligence caused the beautiful human body to exist, and then ran away and left it to its fate, for they know that the Intelligence still presides over each and every function of the body, and may be safely trusted and not feared.

That intelligence, the manifestation of which we call " Nature " or " The Life Principle," and similar names, is constantly on the alert to repair damage, heal wounds, knit together broken bones ; to throw off harmful materials which have accumulated in the system; and in thousands of ways to keep the machine in good running order. Much that we call disease is really a beneficent action of Nature designed to get rid of poisonous substances which we have allowed to enter and remain in our system.

Let us see just what this body means. Let us suppose a soul seeking a tenement in which to work out this phase of its existence. Occultists know that in order to manifest in certain ways the soul has need of a fleshly habitation. Let us see what the soul requires in the way of a body, and then let us see whether Nature has given it what it needs.

In the first place, the soul needs a highly organized physical instrument of thought, and a central station from which it may direct the workings of the body. Nature provides that wonderful instrument, the human brain, the possibilities of which we, at this time, but faintly recognize. The portion of the brain which Man uses in this stage of his development is but a tiny part of the entire brain-area. The unused portion is awaiting the evolution of the race.

Secondly, the soul needs organs designed to receive and record the various forms of impressions from without. Nature steps in and provides the eye, the ear, the nose, the organs of taste and the nerves whereby we feel. Nature is keeping other senses in reserve, until the need of them is felt by the race.

Then, means of communication between the brain and the different parts of the body are needed. Nature has "wired" the body with nerves in a wonderful manner. The brain telegraphs over these wires instructions to all parts of the body, sending its orders to cell and organ, and insisting upon immediate obedience. The brain receives telegrams from all parts of the body, warning it of danger; calling for help; making complaints, etc.

Then the body must have means of moving around in the world. It has outgrown the plant-like inherited tendencies, and wants to "move on." Besides this it wants to reach out after things and turn them to its own use. Nature has provided limbs, and muscles, and tendons, with which to work the limbs.

Then the body needs a framework to keep it in shape, to protect it from shocks; to give it strength and firmness; to prop it up, as it were. Nature gives it the bony frame known as the skeleton, a marvellous piece of machinery, which is well worthy of your study.

The soul needs a physical means of communication with other embodied souls. Nature supplies the means of communication in the organs of speech and hearing.

The body needs a system of carrying repair materials to all of its system, to build up; replenish; repair; and strengthen all the several parts. It also needs a similar system whereby the waste, refuse matter may be carried to the crematory, burned up and sent out of the system. Nature gives us the life-carrying blood—the arteries and veins through which it flows to and fro performing its work—the lungs to oxygenize the blood and to burn up the waste matter.

The body needs material from the outside, with which to build up and repair its parts. Nature provides means of eating the food; of digesting it; of extracting the nutritious elements ; of converting it into shape for absorption by the system ; of excreting the waste portions.

And, finally, the body is provided with means of reproducing its kind, and providing other souls with fleshly tenements.

It is well worth the time of anyone to study something of the wonderful mechanism and workings of the human body. One gets from this study a most convincing realization of the reality of that great Intelligence in nature—he sees the great Life Principle in operation—he sees that it is not blind chance, or haphazard happening, but that it is the work of a mighty INTELLIGENCE.

Then he learns to trust that Intelligence, and to know that that which brought him into physical being will carry him through life—that the power which took charge of him *then*, has charge of him *now*, and will have charge of him *always*.

As we open ourselves to the inflow of the great Life Principle, so will we be benefited. If we fear it, or trust it not, we shut the door upon it and must necessarily suffer.

CHAPTER IV

OUR FRIEND, THE VITAL FORCE

MANY people make the mistake of considering Disease as an entity—a real thing—an opponent of Health. This is incorrect. Health is the natural state of Man, and Disease is simply the absence of Health. If one can comply with the laws of Nature he cannot be sick. When some law is violated, abnormal conditions result, and certain symptoms manifest themselves, and to which symptoms we give the name of some disease. That which we call Disease is simply the result of Nature's attempt to throw off, or dislodge, the abnormal condition, in order to resume normal action.

We are so apt to consider, and speak of, Disease as an entity. We say that "it" attacks us—that "it" seats itself in an organ—that "it" runs its course—that "it" is very malignant—that "it" is quite mild—that "it" persistently resists all treatment—that "it" yields readily—etc., etc. We speak of it as if it were an entity possessed of character, disposition and vital qualities. We consider it as something which takes possession of us and uses its power for our destruction. We speak of it as we would a wolf in a sheepfold—a weasel in the chicken roost—a rat in the granary—and go about fighting it as we would one of the animals above mentioned. We seek to kill it, or at least to scare it away.

Nature is not fickle or unreliable. Life manifests itself within the body in pursuance to well established laws, and pursues its way, slowly, rising until it reaches its zenith, then gradually going down the decline until the time comes for the body to be thrown off like an old, well-used garment, when the soul steps out on its mission of further development. Nature never intended that a man should part with his body until a ripe old age was attained, and the Yogis know that if Nature's laws are observed from childhood, the death of a young or middle aged person from disease would be as rare as is death from accident.

There is within every physical body, a certain vital force which is constantly doing the best it can for us, notwithstanding the reckless way in which we violate the cardinal principles of right living. Much of that which we call disease is but a defensive action of this vital force—a remedial effect. It is not a downward action but an upward action on the part of the living organism. The action is abnormal, because the conditions are abnormal, and the whole recuperative effort of the vital force is exerted toward the restoration of normal conditions.

The first great principle of the Vital Force is *self-preservation.* This principle is ever in evidence, wherever life exists. Under its action the male and female are attracted—the embryo and infant are provided with nourishment—the mother is caused to bear heroically the pains of maternity—the parents are impelled to shelter and protect their offspring under the most adverse circumstances—Why? Because all this means the instinct of *race-preservation.*

But the instinct of preservation of individual life is equally strong. "All that a man hath will he give for his life," saith the writer, and while it is not strictly true of the developed man, it is sufficiently true to use for the purpose of illustrating the principle of self-preservation. And this instinct is not of the Intellect, but is found down among the foundation stones of being. It is an *instinct* which often overrules Intellect. It makes a man's legs "run away with him" when he had firmly resolved to stand in a dangerous position—it causes a shipwrecked man to violate some of the principles of civilization, causing him to kill and eat his comrade and drink his blood—it has made wild beasts of men in the terrible "Black Hole"—and under many and varying conditions it asserts its supremacy. It is working always for life—more life—for health—more health. And it often makes us sick in order to make us healthier—brings on a disease in order to get rid of some foul matter which our carelessness and folly has allowed to intrude in the system.

This principle of self-preservation on the part of the Vital Force, also moves us along in the direction of health, as surely as does the influence within the magnetic needle make it point due north. We may turn aside, not heeding the impulse, but the urge is always there. The same instinct is within us, which, in the seed, causes it to put forth its little shoot, often moving weights a thousand times heavier than itself, in its effort to get to the sunlight. The same impulse causes the sapling to shoot upward from the ground. The same principle causes roots to spread downward and outward. In each case, although the direction is different, each move is in the *right* direction. If we are wounded, the Vital Force begins to heal the wound, doing the work with wonderful sagacity and precision. If we break a bone, all that we, or the surgeon may do, is to place the bones into juxtaposition and keep them there, while the great Vital Force knits the fractured parts together. If we fall, or our muscles or ligaments are torn, all that we can do is to observe certain things in the way of attention, and the Vital Force starts in to do its work, and drawing on the system for the necessary materials, repairs the damage.

All physicians know, and their schools teach, that if a man is in good physical condition, his Vital Force will cause him to recover from almost any condition excepting when the vital organs are destroyed. When the physical system has been allowed to run down, recovery is much more difficult, if, indeed, not impossible, as the efficiency of the Vital Force is impaired and is compelled to work under adverse conditions. But rest assured that it is doing the best it can for you, always, under the existing conditions. If Vital Force cannot do for you all that it aims to do, it will not give up the attempt as hopeless, but will accommodate itself to circumstances and make the best of it. Give it a free hand and it will keep you in perfect health—restrict it by irrational and unnatural methods of living, and it will still try to pull you through, and will serve you until the end, to the best of its ability, in spite of your ingratitude and stupidity. It will fight for you to the finish.

The principle of *accommodation* is manifested all through all forms of life. A seed dropped into the crevice of a rock, when it begins to grow either becomes squeezed into the shape of the rock, or, if it be strong enough, splits the rock in twain and attains its normal shape. So, in the case of Man, who manages to live and thrive in all climates, and conditions, the Vital Force has accommodated itself to the varying conditions, and, where it could not split the rock, it sent out the sprout in a somewhat distorted shape, but still alive and hardy.

No organism can become diseased while the proper conditions for health are observed. Health is but life under normal conditions, while disease is life under abnormal conditions. The conditions which caused a man to grow to a healthy, vigorous manhood are necessary to *keep* him in health and vigour. Given the right condition, the Vital Force will do its best work, but given imperfect conditions the Vital Force will be able to manifest but imperfectly, and more or less of what we call disease ensues. We are living in a civilization which has forced a more or less unnatural mode of life upon us, and the Vital Force finds it hard to do as well for us as it would like. We do not eat naturally; drink naturally; sleep naturally; breathe naturally; or dress naturally. We " have done those things which we ought not to have done, and we have left undone those things which we ought to have done, and there is no Health within us "—or, we might add, as little health as we can help.

We have dwelt upon the matter of the friendliness of the Vital Force, for the reason that it is a matter usually overlooked by those who have not made a study of it. It forms a part of the Yogi Philosophy of Hatha Yoga, and the Yogis take it largely into consideration in their lives. They know that they have a good friend and a strong ally in the Vital Force, and they allow it to flow freely through them, and try to interfere as little as possible with its operations. They know that the Vital Force is ever awake to their well-being and health, and they repose the greatest confidence in it.

Much of the success of Hatha Yoga consists of methods best calculated to allow the Vital Force to work freely and without hindrance, and its methods and exercises are largely devoted to that end. To clear the track of obstructions, and to give the chariot of the Vital Force the right of way on a smooth, clear road, is the aim of the Hatha Yogi. Follow his precepts and it will be well with your body.

CHAPTER V

THE LABORATORY OF THE BODY

This little book is not intended for a text-book upon physiology, but inasmuch as the majority of people seem to have little or no idea of the nature, functions and uses of the various bodily organs, we think it as well to say a few words regarding the very important organs of the body which have to do with the digestion and assimilation of the food which nourishes the body—which perform the laboratory work of the system.

The first bit of the human machinery of digestion to be considered by us are the teeth. Nature has provided us with teeth to bite our food and grind it into fine bits, thus rendering it of a convenient size and consistency to be easily acted upon by the saliva and the digestive juices of the stomach, after which it is reduced to a liquid form that its nourishing qualities may be easily assimilated and absorbed by the body. This seems to be merely a repetition of an oft-told tale, but how many of our readers really act as if they knew for what purpose their teeth had been given them? They bolt their food just as if teeth were merely for show, and generally act as if Nature had provided them with a gizzard, by the aid of which they could like the fowl grind up and break into small bits the food that they had bolted. Remember, friends, that your teeth were given you for a purpose, and also consider the fact that if Nature had intended you to bolt your food she would have provided you with a gizzard instead of with teeth. We will have much to say about the proper use of the teeth as we go along, as it has a very close connection with a vital principle of Hatha Yoga, as you will see after a while.

The next organs to be considered are the Salivary Glands. These glands are six in number, of which four are located under the tongue and jaw, and two in the cheeks in the front of the ears, one on each side. Their best known function is to manufacture, generate or secrete saliva, which, when needed, flows out through numerous ducts in different parts of the mouth, and mixes with the food which is being chewed or masticated. The food being chewed into small particles, the saliva is able to more thoroughly reach all portions of it with a correspondingly increased effect. The saliva moistens the food, thus allowing it to be more easily swallowed, this function, however, being a mere incident to its more important ones. Its best known function (and the one which Western science teaches is its most important one) is its chemical offices, which convert the starchy food matter into sugar, thus performing the first step in the process of digestion.

Here is another oft-told tale. You all know about the saliva, but how many of you eat in a manner which allows Nature to put the saliva to work as she had designed? You bolt your food after a few perfunctory chews and defeat Nature's plans, toward which she has gone to so much trouble, and to perform which she has built such beautiful and delicate machinery. But Nature manages to "get back" at you for your contempt and disregard of her plans—Nature has a good memory and always makes you pay your debts.

We must not forget to mention the tongue—that faithful friend who is so often made to perform the ignoble task of assisting in the utterance of angry words, retailing of gossip, lying, nagging, swearing, and last but not least, complaining.

The tongue has a most important work to perform in the process of nourishing the body with food. Besides a number of mechanical movements which it performs in eating, in which it helps to move the food along and its similar service in the act of swallowing, it is the organ of taste and passes critical judgment upon the food which asks admittance to the stomach.

You have neglected the normal uses of the teeth, the salivary glands and the tongue, and they have consequently failed to give you the best service. If you but trust them and return to sane and normal methods of eating you will find them gladly and cheerfully responding to your trust and will once more give you their full share of service. They are good friends and servants, but need a little confidence, trust and responsibility to bring out their best points.

After the food has been chewed or masticated and then saturated with saliva it passes down the throat into the stomach. The lower part of the throat, which is called the gullet, performs a peculiar muscular contraction, which pushes downward the particles of food, which act forms a part of the process of "swallowing." The process of converting the starchy portion of the food into sugar, or glucose, which is begun by the saliva in the mouth, is continued as the food passes into and down the gullet, but nearly, or entirely ceases, when the food once reaches the stomach, which fact must be considered when one studies the subject of the advantage of a deliberate habit of eating, as, if the food is hastily chewed and swallowed, it reaches the stomach only partially affected by the saliva and in an imperfect condition for Nature's subsequent work.

The stomach itself is a pear-shaped bag with a capacity of about one quart or more in some cases. The food enters the stomach from the gullet on the upper left-hand side, just below the heart. The food afterwards leaves the stomach on the lower right-hand and enters the small intestine by means of a peculiar sort of valve, which is so wonderfully constructed that it allows the matter from the stomach to pass easily through it, but refuses to allow anything to work back from the intestine into the stomach. This valve is known as the "Pyloric Valve" or the "Pyloric Orifice," the word "Pyloric" being derived from the Greek word which means "gatekeeper"—and indeed this little valve acts as a most intelligent gatekeeper, always on the watch, never asleep.

The stomach is a great chemical laboratory in which the food undergoes chemical changes which allow it to be taken up by the system and changed into a nourishing material which is converted into rich, red blood which courses all over the body, building up, repairing, strengthening and adding to all the parts and organs.

The "inside" of the stomach is covered with a lining of delicate mucous membrane, which is filled with minute glands, all of which open into the stomach and around which is a very fine network of minute blood-vessels with remarkably thin walls, from which is manufactured, or secreted, that wonderful fluid, the gastric juice. The gastric juice is a powerful liquid acting as a solvent upon what is called the nitrogenous portions of the food. It also acts upon the sugar or glucose which has been manufactured from the starchy food by the saliva, as above described. It is a bitter sort of liquid, containing a chemical product called pepsin, which is its active agent and which plays a most important part in the digestion of the food.

In a normal, healthy person the stomach manufactures or secretes about one gallon of gastric juice in twenty-four hours, and uses same in the process of digestion of the food. When the food reaches the stomach the little glands, before mentioned, pour out a sufficient supply of the gastric juice, which mixes up with the mass of food in the stomach. Then the stomach sets up sort of a churning motion, which moves the pulpy food round and round, from end to end, from side to side, twisting and turning it, churning and kneading it, until the gastric juice penetrates every part of the mass and is well mixed up into it. The Instinctive Mind does some wonderful work in the stomach movements and works like a well oiled machine.

And if the stomach has been treated to properly

prepared, well chewed food, properly insalivated, the machine is able to turn out a fine job. But if, as so often happens, the food is of a quality not fit for the human stomach—or if it has been but half chewed, or bolted—or if the stomach has been "stuffed" by a gluttonous owner—there is going to be trouble. In such a case, instead of the normal process of digestion being performed, the stomach is unable to do its work and *fermentation* results, and the stomach becomes the holder of a fermenting, putrefying, rotting mass—a "yeast pot" it has been called under such circumstances. If people could but form an idea of what a cesspool they maintain in their stomachs they would cease to shrug their shoulders and look bored whenever the subject of rational and sane habits of eating are mentioned.

This putrefying ferment, arising from abnormal habits of eating, often becomes chronic and results in a condition which manifests itself in the symptoms of what is called "dyspepsia," or similar troubles. It remains in the stomach for a long time after the meal, and then when the next meal reaches the stomach the fermentation continues until the stomach actually becomes a perpetually active "yeast pot." This condition, of course, results in an impairment of the normal functioning of the stomach, the surface of which becomes slimy, soft, thin and weak. The glands become clogged and the whole digestive apparatus of the stomach becomes impaired and broken down. In such event the half digested food passes out into the small intestine, tainted with the acids arising from fermentation, and the result is that the whole system becomes gradually poisoned and imperfectly nourished.

The food-mass saturated with the gastric juice which has been poured upon it and kneaded and churned into it, leaves the stomach by the Pyloric orifice on the lower right-hand side of the stomach, and enters the small intestine.

The small intestine is a tube-like canal ingeniously coiled upon itself so as to occupy but a comparatively small space, but which is really from twenty to thirty feet in length. Its inner walls are lined with a velvety substance, and through the greater part of its length this velvety lining is arranged in transverse shelf-like folds, which maintain a sort of "winking" motion, swaying backward and forward in the intestinal fluids, retarding the passage of the food and providing an increased surface for secretion and absorption. The velvety condition of this mucous lining is caused by numerous minute elevations, something like the surface of a piece of plush, which are known as the intestinal "villi," the office of which will be explained a little further on.

As soon as the food-mass enters the small intestine it is met with a peculiar fluid called the bile, which saturates it and is thoroughly mixed up with it. The bile is a secretion of the liver and is stored up ready for use in a strong bag, known as the gall bladder. About two quarts of bile per day is used in saturating the food as it passes into the small intestine. Its purpose is to assist the pancreatic juice in preparing the fatty parts of the food for absorption and also to aid in the prevention of decomposition and putrefaction of the food as it passes through the small intestine and the neutralization of the gastric juice which has already performed its work. The pancreatic juice is secreted by the pancreas, an elongated organ situated just behind the stomach, and its purpose is to act upon the fatty portions of the food and to render them possible of absorption from the intestines along with the other parts of the food nourishment. About one and one-half pints is used daily in this work.

The hundreds of thousands of plush-like " hairs " upon the velvety lining of the small intestine (above alluded to), and which are known as " villi," maintain a constant waving motion, passing through and in the soft, semi-liquid food which is passing through the small intestine. They are constantly in motion, licking up and absorbing the nourishment that is contained in the food-mass and transmitting it to the system.

The several steps whereby the food is converted into blood and is carried to all parts of the system are as follows: Mastication, insalivation, deglutition, stomach and intestinal digestion, absorption, circulation and assimilation. Let us run over them again hastily that we may not forget them.

Mastication is performed by the teeth—it is the chewing process—the lips, tongue and cheeks assisting in the work. It breaks up the food into small particles and enables the saliva to reach it more thoroughly.

Insalivation is the process of saturating the masticated food with the saliva which pours into it from the salivary glands. The saliva acts upon the cooked starch in the food, changing it into dextrine and then into glucose, thus rendering it soluble. This chemical change is rendered possible by the action of the pytaline in the saliva acting as a ferment and changing the chemical constitution of those substances for which it has an affinity.

Digestion is performed in the stomach and small intestines and consists in the conversion of the food-mass into products capable of being absorbed and assimilated. Digestion begins when the food reaches the stomach. The gastric juice then pours out copiously, and, becoming mixed up with and churned into the food-mass, it dissolves the connective tissue of meat, releases fat from its envelopes by breaking them up and transforms some of the albuminous material, such as lean meat, the gluten of wheat and white of eggs, into albuminose, in which form they are capable of being absorbed and assimilated. The transformation occasioned by stomach digestion is accomplished by the chemical action of an organic ingredient of the gastric juice, called pepsin, in connection with the acid ingredients of the gastric juice.

While the process of digestion is being performed by the stomach the fluid portion of the food-mass, both that which has entered the stomach as fluids which have been drunken, as well as the fluids liberated from the solid food in the process of digestion, is rapidly taken up by the absorbents of the stomach and is carried to the blood, while the more solid portions of the food-mass are churned up by the muscular action of the stomach, as we have stated. In about a half-hour the solid portions of the food-mass begin slowly to leave the stomach in the form of a grayish, pasty substance, called chyme, which is a mixture of some of the sugar and salts of the food, of transformed starch or glucose, of softened starch, of broken fat and connective tissue, and of albuminose.

The chyme, leaving the stomach, enters the small intestine, as we have described, and comes in contact with the pancreatic and intestinal juices and with the bile, and intestinal digestion ensues. These fluids dissolve most of the food that has not already been softened. Intestinal digestion resolves the chyme into three substances, known as (1) Peptone, from the digestion of albuminous particles; (2) Chyle, from the emulsion of the fats; (3) Glucose, from the transformation of the starchy elements of the food. These substances are, to a large extent, carried into the blood and become a part of it, while the undigested food passes out of the small intestine through a trap-door-like valve into the large bowel called the colon, of which we shall speak by-and-by.

Absorption, by which name is known the process by which the above-named products of the food, resulting from the digestive process, are taken up by the veins and lacteals, is effected by endosmosis. The water and the fluids liberated from the food-mass by the stomach digestion are rapidly absorbed and carried away by the blood in the portal vein to the liver. The peptone and glucose from the small intestines also reaches the portal vein to the liver through the blood-vessels of the intestinal villi, which we have described. This blood reaches the heart after passing through the liver, where it undergoes a process which we will speak of when we reach the subject of the liver. The chyle, which is the remaining product of the food-mass in the intestines after the peptone and glucose have been taken up and carried to the liver, is taken up and passes through the lacteals into the thoracic duct, and is gradually conveyed to the blood, as will be further described in our chapter on the Circulation. In our chapter on the Circulation we will explain how the blood carries the nutriment derived from the digested food to all parts of the body, giving to each tissue, cell, organ and part the material by which it builds up and repairs itself, thus enabling the body to grow and develop.

The liver secretes the bile, which is carried to the small intestine, as we have stated. It also stores up a substance called glycogen, which is formed in the liver from the digested materials brought to it by the portal vein (as above explained). Glycogen is stored up in the liver, and is afterwards gradually transformed, in the intervals of digestion, into glucose or a substance similar to grape sugar. The pancreas secretes the pancreatic juices, which it pours into the small intestine, to aid in intestinal digestion, where it acts chiefly upon the fatty portions of the food. The kidneys are located in the loins, behind the intestines. They are two in number and are shaped like beans. They purify the blood by removing from it a poisonous substance called urea and other waste products. The fluid secreted by the kidneys is carried by two tubes, called ureters, to the bladder. The bladder is located in the pelvis and serves as a reservoir for the urine, which consists of waste fluids carrying with it refuse matter of the system.

Before leaving this part of the subject we wish to call the attention of our readers to the fact that when the food enters the stomach and small intestines improperly masticated and insalivated—when the teeth and salivary glands have not been given a chance to do their work properly—digestion is interfered with and impeded and the digestive organs are overworked and are rendered unable to accomplish what is asked of them. It is like asking one set of workmen to do their own work in addition to the work which should have been previously performed by another set of men—it is asking the railroad engineer to perform the duties of fireman as well as his own—to keep the fire going on an up grade and run the locomotive on a dangerous bit of road at the same time. The absorbents of the stomach and intestines must absorb *something*—that is their business—and if you do not give them the proper materials they will absorb the fermenting and putrefying mass in the stomach and pass it along to the blood. The blood carries this poor material to all parts of the body, including the brain, and it is no wonder that people complain of biliousness, headache, etc., when they are being self-poisoned in this way.

CHAPTER VI

THE LIFE FLUID

In our last chapter we gave you an idea of how the food we eat is gradually transformed and resolved into substances capable of being absorbed and taken up by the blood, which carries the nourishment to all parts of the system, where it is used in building up, repairing and renewing the several parts of the physical man. In this chapter we will give you a brief description of how this work of the blood is carried on.

The nutritive portion of the digested food is taken up by the circulation and becomes blood. The blood flows through the arteries to every cell and tissue of the body that it may perform its constructive and recuperative work. It then returns through the arteries, carrying with it the broken-down cells and other waste matter of the system, that the waste may be expelled from the system by the lungs and other organs performing the "casting-out" work of the system. This flow of the blood to and from the heart is called the Circulation.

The engine which drives this wonderful system of physical machinery is, of course, the Heart. We will not take up your time describing the heart, but will instead tell you something of the work performed by it.

Let us begin at the point at which we left off in our

last chapter—the point at which the nourishment of the food, taken up by the blood which assimilates it, reaches the heart, which sends it out on its errand of nourishing the body.

The blood starts on its journey through the arteries, which are a series of elastic canals, having divisions and subdivisions, beginning with the main canals which feed the smaller ones, which in turn feed still smaller ones until the capillaries are reached. The capillaries are very small blood-vessels measuring about one three-thousandth of an inch in diameter. They resemble very fine hairs, which resemblance gives them their name. The capillaries penetrate the tissues in meshes of network, bringing the blood in close contact with all the parts. Their walls are very thin and the nutritious ingredients of the blood exude through their walls and are taken up by the tissues. The capillaries not only exude the nourishment from the blood, but they also take up the blood on its return journey (as we will see presently) and generally fetch and carry for the system, including the absorption of the nourishment of the food from the intestinal villi, as described in our last chapter.

Well, to get back to the arteries. They carry the rich, red, pure blood from the heart, laden with health-giving nutrition and life, distributing it through large canals into smaller, from smaller into still smaller, until finally the tiny hair-like capillaries are reached and the tissues take up the nourishment and use it for building purposes, the wonderful little cells of the body doing this work most intelligently. (We shall have something to say regarding the work of these cells, by-and-by.) The blood having given up a supply of nourishment, begins its return journey to the heart, taking with it the waste products, dead cells, broken-down tissue and other refuse of the system. It starts with the capillaries, but this return journey is not made through the arteries, but by a switch-off arrangement it is directed into the smaller veinlets of the venous system (or system of veins"), from whence it passes to the larger veins and on to the heart. Before it reaches the arteries again, on a new trip, however, something happens to it. It goes to the crematory of the lungs, in order to have its waste matter and impurities burnt up and cast off. In another chapter we will tell you about this work of the lungs.

Before passing on, however, we must tell you that there exists another fluid which circulates through the system. This is called the Lymph, which closely resembles the blood in composition. It contains some of the ingredients of the blood which have exuded from the walls of the blood-vessels and some of the waste products of the system, which, after being cleansed and "made-over" by the lymphatic system, re-enter the blood, and are again used. The lymph circulates in thin vein-like canals, so small that they cannot be readily seen by the human eye, until they are injected with quicksilver. These canals empty into several of the large veins, and the lymph then mingles with the returning blood, on its way to the heart. The "Chyle," after leaving the small intestine (see last lesson) mingles with the lymph from the lower parts of the body, and gets into the blood in this way, while the other products of the digested food pass through the portal vein and the liver on their journey—so that, although they take different routes, they meet again in the circulating blood.

So, you will see, the blood is the constituent of the body which, directly or indirectly, furnishes nourishment and life to all the parts of the body. If the blood is poor, or the circulation weak, nutrition of some parts of the body must be impaired, and diseased conditions will result. The blood supplies about one-tenth of man's weight. Of this amount about one-quarter is distributed in the heart, lungs, large arteries and veins; about one-quarter in the liver; about one-quarter in the muscles, the remaining quarter being distributed among the remaining organs and tissues. The brain utilizes about one-fifth of the entire quantity of blood.

Remember, always, in thinking about the blood, that the blood is what you make it by the food you eat, and the way you eat it. You can have the very best kind of blood, and plenty of it, by selecting the proper foods, and by eating such food as Nature intended you to do. Or, on the other hand, you may have very poor blood, and an insufficient quantity of it, by foolish gratification of the abnormal Appetite, and by improper eating (not worthy of the name) of any kind of food. The blood is the life—and you make the blood—that is the matter in a nutshell.

Now, let us pass on to the crematory of the lungs, and see what is going to happen to that blue, impure venous blood, which has come back from all parts of the body, laden with impurities and waste matter. Let us have a look at the crematory.

CHAPTER VII

THE CREMATORY OF THE SYSTEM

THE Organs of Respiration consist of the lungs and the air passages leading to them. The lungs are two in number, and occupy the pleural chamber of the thorax, one on each side of the median line, being separated from each other by the heart, the greater blood-vessels and the larger air tubes. Each lung is free in all directions, except at the root, which consists chiefly of the bronchi, arteries and veins connecting the lungs with the trachea and heart. The lungs are spongy and porous, and their tissues are very elastic. They are covered with a delicately constructed but strong sac, known as the pleural sac, one wall of which closely adheres to the lung, and the other to the inner wall of the chest, and which secretes a fluid which allows the inner surfaces of the walls to glide easily upon each other in the act of breathing.

The Air Passages consist of the interior of the nose, pharynx, larynx, windpipe or trachea, and the bronchial tubes. When we breathe, we draw in the air through the nose, in which it is warmed by contact with the mucous membrane, which is richly supplied with blood, and after it has passed through the pharynx and larynx it passes into the trachea or windpipe, which subdivides into numerous tubes called the bronchial tubes (bronchia), which, in turn, subdivide into and terminate in minute subdivisions in all the small air spaces in the lungs, of which the lungs contain millions. A writer has stated that if the air cells of the lungs were spread out over an unbroken surface, they would cover an area of fourteen thousand square feet.

The air is drawn into the lungs by the action of the diaphragm, a great, strong, flat, sheet-like muscle, stretched across the chest, separating the chest-box from the abdomen. The diaphragm's action is almost as automatic as that of the heart, although it may be transformed into a semi-voluntary muscle by an effort of the will. When it expands, it increases the size of the chest and lungs, and the air rushes into the vacuum thus created. When it relaxes, the chest and lungs contract and the air is expelled from the lungs.

Now, before considering what happens to the air in the lungs, let us look a little into the matter of the circulation of the blood. The blood, as you know, is driven by the heart, through the arteries, into the capillaries, thus reaching every part of the body, which it vitalizes, nourishes and strengthens. It then returns by means of the capillaries by another route, the veins, to the heart, from whence it is drawn to the lungs.

The blood starts on its arterial journey, bright red and rich, laden with life-giving qualities and properties. It returns by the venous route, poor, blue and dull, being laden down with the waste matter of the system. It goes out like a fresh stream from the mountains; it returns as a stream of sewer water. This foul stream goes to the right auricle of the heart. When this auricle becomes filled, it contracts and forces the stream of blood through an opening in the right ventricle of the heart, which in turn sends it on to the lungs, where it is distributed by millions of hair-like blood-vessels to the air cells of the lungs, of which we have spoken. Now, let us take up the story of the lungs at this point.

The foul stream of blood is now distributed among the millions of tiny air cells in the lungs. A breath of air is inhaled and the oxygen of the air comes in contact with the impure blood through the thin walls of the hair-like blood-vessels of the lungs, which walls are thick enough to hold the blood, but thin enough to admit the oxygen to penetrate them. When the oxygen comes in contact with the blood, a form of combustion takes place, and the blood takes up oxygen and releases carbonic acid gas generated from the waste products and poisonous matter which has been gathered up by the blood from all parts of the system. The blood thus purified and oxygenated is carried back to the heart, again rich, red and bright, and laden with life-giving properties and qualities. Upon reaching the left auricle of the heart, it is forced into the left ventricle, from whence it is again forced out through the arteries on its mission of life to all parts of the system. It is estimated that in a single day of twenty-four hours, 35,000 pints of blood traverse the capillaries of the lungs, the blood corpuscles passing in single file and being exposed to the oxygen of the air on both of their surfaces. When one considers the minute details of the process alluded to, he is lost in wonder and admiration at Nature's infinite care and intelligence.

It will be seen that unless fresh air in sufficient

quantities reaches the lungs, the foul stream of venous blood cannot be purified, and consequently not only is the body thus robbed of nourishment, but the waste products which should have been destroyed are returned to the circulation and poison the system, and death ensues. Impure air acts in the same way, only in a lessened degree. It will also be seen that if one does not breathe in a sufficient quantity of air, the work of the blood cannot go on properly, and the result is that the body is insufficiently nourished and disease ensues, or a state of imperfect health is experienced. The blood of one who breathes improperly is, of course, of a bluish, dark colour, lacking the rich redness of pure arterial blood. This often shows itself in a poor complexion. Proper breathing, and a consequent good circulation, results in a clear, bright complexion.

A little reflection will show the vital importance of Correct breathing. If the blood is not fully purified by the regenerative process of the lungs, it returns to the arteries in an abnormal state, insufficiently purified and imperfectly cleansed of the impurities which it took up on its return journey. These impurities if returned to the system will certainly manifest in some form of disease, either in a form of blood disease or some disease resulting from impaired functioning of some insufficiently nourished organ or tissue.

The blood, when properly exposed to the air in the lungs, not only has its impurities consumed, and parts with its noxious carbonic acid gas, but it also takes up and absorbs a certain quantity of oxygen which it carries to all parts of the body, where it is needed in order that Nature may perform her processes properly. When the oxygen comes in contact with the blood, it unites with the hæmoglobin of the blood and is carried to every cell, tissue, muscle and organ, which it invigorates and strengthens, replacing the worn-out cells and tissue by new materials which Nature converts to her use. Arterial blood, properly exposed to the air, contains about 25 per cent. of free oxygen.

Not only is every part vitalized by the oxygen, but the act of digestion depends materially upon a certain amount of oxygenation of the food, and this is only accomplished by the oxygen in the blood coming in contact with the food and producing a certain form of combustion. It is therefore necessary that a proper supply of oxygen be taken through the lungs. This accounts for the fact that weak lungs and poor digestion are so often found together. To grasp the full significance of this statement, one must remember that the entire body receives nourishment from the food assimilated, and that imperfect assimilation always means an imperfectly nourished body. Even the lungs themselves depend upon the same source for nourishment, and if through imperfect breathing the assimilation becomes imperfect, and the lungs in turn become weakened, they are rendered still less able to perform their work properly, and so in turn the body becomes further weakened. Every particle of food and drink must be oxygenated before it can yield us the proper nourishment, and before the waste products of the system can be reduced to the proper condition to be eliminated from the system. Lack of sufficient oxygen means imperfect nutrition, imperfect elimination, and imperfect health. Verily, " breath is life."

The combustion arising from the change in the waste products generates heat and equalizes the temperature of the body. Good breathers are not apt to " take cold," and they generally have plenty of good warm blood which enables them to resist the changes in the outer temperature.

In addition to the above-mentioned important processes, the act of breathing gives exercise to the internal organs and muscles, which feature is generally overlooked by the Western writers on the subject, but which the Yogis fully appreciate.

In imperfect or shallow breathing, only a portion of the lung cells are brought into play, and a great portion of the lung capacity is lost, the system suffering in proportion to the amount of under-oxygenation. The lower animals, in their native state, breathe naturally, and primitive man undoubtedly did the same. The abnormal manner of living adopted by civilized man—the shadow that follows upon civilization—has robbed us of our natural habit of breathing, and the race has greatly suffered thereby. Man's only physical salvation is to " get back to Nature."

CHAPTER VIII

NOURISHMENT

THE human body is constantly undergoing change. Atoms of bone, tissue, flesh, muscle, fat and fluids are constantly being worn out and removed from the system, and new atoms are constantly being manufactured in the wonderful laboratory of the body, and then sent to take the place of the worn-out and discarded material.

Let us consider the physical body of man and its mechanism, as a plant—and, indeed, it is akin to the life of the plant in its nature. What does the plant require to bring it up from seed to sprout, from sprout to plant, with flower, seed and fruit? The answer is simple—fresh air, sunlight, water, and nourishing soil—these things, and all of them, must it have in order to grow to healthy maturity. And Man's physical body requires just the same things—all of them—in order to be healthy, strong and normal. Remember the requisites—fresh air, sunlight, water and food. We will consider the matter of air, sunlight and water in other chapters, and will consider the matter of nourishing food first.

Just as the plant grows slowly, but steadily, so does this great work of discarding worn-out material and the substitution of new material go on constantly, day and night. We are not conscious of this mighty work, as it belongs to that great sub-conscious part of Man's nature—it is a part of the work of the Instinctive Mind.

The whole of the body, and all its parts, depend for

health, strength and vigour upon this constant renewal of material. If this renewal were stopped disintegration and death would ensue. The replacing of the worn-out and discarded material is an imperative necessity of our organism, and, therefore, is the first thing to be considered when we think of the Healthy Man.

The keynote of this subject of food in the Hatha Yoga Philosophy is the Sanscrit word, the English equivalent of which is "NOURISHMENT." We print the word in capital letters that it may make an impression upon your minds. We wish our students to associate the thought of Food with the thought of Nourishment.

To the Yogi, food does not mean something to tickle the abnormal palate, but instead it means, first, *Nourishment*; second, NOURISHMENT, and third, NOURISHMENT. Nourishment first, last and always.

To many of the Western people, the ideal Yogi is a lean, lank, scrawny, half-starved, emaciated being, who thinks so little of food that he goes for days without eating—one who considers food to be too "material" for his "spiritual nature." Nothing can be further from the truth. The Yogis, at least those who are well-grounded in Hatha Yoga, regard Nourishment as his first duty towards his body, and he is always careful to keep that body properly nourished, and to see that the supply of new, fresh material is always at least equal to the worn-out and discarded matter.

It is quite true that the Yogi is not a gross eater, nor is he inclined to rich and fancy dishes. On the contrary, he smiles at the folly of such things, and goes to his plain and nourishing meal, knowing that he will obtain there full nourishment without the waste and harmful matter contained in the more elaborate dishes of his brother who is ignorant of the real meaning of food.

A maxim of Hatha Yoga is: " It is not what a man *eats*, but the amount that he *assimilates*, that nourishes him." There is a world of wisdom in this old maxim, and it contains that which writers upon health subjects have taken volumes to express.

We will show you, later on, the Yogi method of extracting the maximum amount of nourishment from the minimum amount of food. The Yogi method lies in the middle of the road, the two opposite sides of which road are travelled, respectively, by the two differing Western schools, namely the " food-stuffers " and " starvationists," each of whom loudly proclaim the merits of their own cult and decry the claims of the opposing sect. The simple Yogi may be pardoned for smiling good-naturedly at the disputes raging between those who, preaching the necessity of sufficient nutrition, teach that " stuffing " is necessary to obtain it, on the one hand; and at those of the opposing school, who, recognizing the folly of " stuffing " and over-eating, have no remedy to offer but a semi-starvation, accompanied with long continued fasts, which, of course, has brought many of its followers down to weakened bodies, impaired vitality, and even death.

To the Yogi, the evils of malnutrition, on the one hand, and over-eating on the other, do not exist—these questions have been settled for him centuries ago by the old Yogi fathers, whose very names have been almost forgotten by their followers of to-day.

Remember, now, please, once and for all, that Hatha Yoga does not advocate the plan of starving oneself, but, on the contrary, knows and teaches that no human body can be strong and healthy unless it is properly nourished by sufficient food eaten and assimilated. Many delicate, weak and nervous people owe their impaired vitality and diseased condition to the fact that they do not obtain sufficient nourishment.

Remember, also, that Hatha Yoga rejects as ridiculous the theory that Nourishment is obtained from "stuffing," gorging, or over-eating, and views with wonder and pity these attributes of the glutton, and sees nothing in these practices but the manifestation of the attributes of the unclean swine, utterly unworthy of the developed man.

To the Yogi understanding Man should eat to live—not live to eat.

The Yogi is an epicure, rather than a gourmand, for while eating the plainest food he has cultivated and encouraged his natural and normal taste so that his hunger imparts to these simple viands a relish sought after, but not obtained, by those who hunt after rich and expensive triumphs of the *chef*. While eating for Nourishment as his main object, he manages to make his food yield him a pleasure unknown to his brother who scorns the simple fare.

In our next chapter we will take up the subject of Hunger and Appetite—two entirely different attributes of the physical body, although to most persons the two appear to mean almost the same thing.

CHAPTER IX

HUNGER VS. APPETITE

As we said at the conclusion of the preceding chapter, Hunger and Appetite are two entirely different attributes of the human body. Hunger is the normal demand for food—Appetite the abnormal craving. Hunger is like the rosy hue upon the cheek of the healthy child—Appetite is like the rouged face of the woman of fashion. And yet most people use the terms as if their meaning were identical. Let us see wherein lies the difference.

It is quite difficult to explain the respective sensations, or symptoms, of Hunger and Appetite, to the average person who has attained the age of maturity, for the majority of persons of that age have had their natural taste, or hunger-instinct, perverted by Appetite to such an extent that they have not experienced the sensation of genuine hunger for many years, and have forgotten just what it felt like. And it is hard to describe a sensation unless one can call up in the mind of his hearer the recollection of the same, or a similar sensation, experienced at some time in the past. We can describe a sound to the person of normal hearing by comparing it with something he has heard—but imagine the difficulty of conveying an intelligent idea of a sound to a man who was born "stone-deaf"; or of describing a colour to a man born blind; or of giving an intelligent description of an odour to one born without the sense of smell.

To one who has emancipated himself from the thrall of appetite, the respective sensations of Hunger and Appetite are quite different and readily distinguished one from the other, and the mind of such a one readily grasps the precise meaning of each term. But to the ordinary "civilized" man "Hunger" means the source of appetite and "Appetite" the result of hunger. Both words are misused. We must illustrate this by familiar examples.

Let us take Thirst, for instance. All of us know the sensation of a good, natural thirst, which calls for a draught of cool water. It is felt in the mouth and throat, and can be satisfied only with that which Nature intended for it—cool water. Now, this natural thirst is akin to natural Hunger.

How different is this natural thirst from the craving which one acquires for sweetened, flavoured soda-water, ice-cream soda, ginger ale, "pop," "soft drinks," etc., etc. And how different from the thirst (?) which one feels for beer, alcoholic liquors, etc., after the taste has once been acquired. Do you begin to see what we mean?

We hear people say that they are "so thirsty" for a glass of soda-water; or others say that they are "thirsty" for a drink of whisky. Now, if these people were really thirsty, or, in other words, if Nature was really calling for fluids, pure water would be just what they would first seek for, and pure water would be the thing which would best gratify the thirst. But, no! water will not satisfy this soda-water or whisky thirst. Why? Simply because it is a craving of an appetite which is not a natural thirst, but which is, on the contrary, an abnormal appetite—a perverted taste. The appetite has been created—the habit acquired—and it is asserting the mastery. You will notice that the victims of these abnormal "thirsts" will occasionally experience a *real* thirst, at which time water alone will be sought, and the tipple of the appetite not thought of. Just think a moment—is not this so with you? This is not a lecture directed against the fancy drink habit, or a temperance sermon, but just an illustration of the difference between a natural instinct and an acquired habit, or appetite. Appetite is an acquired habit of eating or drinking, and has but little to do with real hunger or thirst.

A man acquires an appetite for tobacco in any of its forms; or for liquor, or for chewing-gum, or for opium, morphine, cocaine, or similar drugs. And an appetite once acquired becomes, if anything, stronger than that natural demand for food or drink, for men have been known to die of starvation because they had spent all of their money for drink or narcotics. Men have sold their babies' stockings for drink—have stolen and even murdered in order to gratify their appetite for narcotics. And yet who would think of calling this terrible craving of appetite by the name of Hunger? And yet we continue to speak of, and think of, every craving for something to put into the stomach as Hunger, while many of these cravings are as much a symptom of Appetite as is the craving or desire for alcohol or narcotics.

The lower animal has a natural hunger until it is spoiled by contact with man (or woman) who tempts it with candies and similar articles, miscalled food. The young child has a natural hunger until it is spoiled in the same way. In the child, natural hunger is more or less replaced by acquired appetites, the degree depending largely upon the amount of wealth its parents possess—the greater the wealth, the greater the acquirement of false appetite. And as it grows older, it loses all recollection of what real Hunger means. In fact, people speak of Hunger as a distressing thing, rather than as a natural instinct. Sometimes men go out camping, and the open air, exercise, and natural life gives them again a taste of real hunger, and they eat like school boys and with a relish they have not known for years. They feel "hungry" in earnest, and eat because they have to, not from mere habit, as they do when they are home and are overloading their stomachs continually.

We recently read of a party of wealthy people who were shipwrecked while on a yachting pleasure trip. They were compelled to live on the most meagre fare for about ten days. When rescued they looked the picture of health—rosy, bright-eyed, and possessed of the precious gift of a good, natural Hunger. Some of the party had been dyspeptics for years, but the ten days' experience with food scarce and at a premium, had completely cured them of their dyspepsia and other troubles. They had obtained sufficient to properly nourish them, and had gotten rid of the waste products of the system which had been poisoning them. Whether or not they "stayed cured" depended upon whether they again exchanged Hunger for Appetite.

Natural Hunger—like natural Thirst—expresses itself through the nerves of the mouth and throat. When one is hungry, the thought or mention of food causes a peculiar sensation in the mouth, throat and salivary glands. The nerves of those parts manifest a peculiar sensation, the saliva begins to flow, and the whole of the region manifests a desire to get to work. The stomach gives no symptoms whatever, and is not at all in evidence at such times. One feels that the "taste" of good wholesome food would be most pleasurable. There is none of those feelings of faintness, emptiness, gnawing, "all-goneness," etc., in the region of the stomach. These last mentioned symptoms are all characteristic of the Appetite habit, which is insisting that the habit must be continued. Did you ever notice that the drink habit calls forth just such symptoms? The craving and "all-gone" feeling is characteristic of both forms of abnormal appetite. The man who is craving a smoke, or a chew of tobacco feels the same way.

A man often wonders why he cannot get a dinner such as "mother used to cook." Do you know why he cannot get it? Simply because he has replaced his natural Hunger by an abnormal appetite, and he does not feel satisfied unless he gratifies that Appetite, which renders the homely fare of the past an impossibility. If the man were to cultivate a natural hunger, by a return to first principles, he would have restored to him the meals of his youth—he would find many cooks just as good as "mother" was, for he would be a boy again.

You are probably wondering what all this has to do with Hatha Yoga, are you not? Well, just this: The Yogi has conquered appetite, and allows Hunger to manifest through him. He enjoys every mouthful of food, even to the crust of dry bread, and obtains nourishment and pleasure from it. He eats it in a manner unknown to most of you, which will be described a little further on, and so far from being a half-starved anchorite, he is a well-fed, properly nourished enjoyer of the feast, for he has possessed himself of that most piquant of all sauces—Hunger.

CHAPTER X

THE YOGI THEORY AND PRACTICE OF PRANA ABSORPTION FROM FOOD

NATURE'S shrewdness in combining several duties into one, and also in rendering necessary duties pleasant (and thereby likely to be performed) is illustrated in numberless ways. One of the most striking examples of this kind will be brought out in this chapter. We will see how she manages to accomplish several things at the same time, and how she also renders pleasant several most necessary offices of the physical system.

Let us start with the statement of the Yogi theory of the absorption of Prana from food. This theory holds that there is contained in the food of man and the lower animals, a certain form of Prana which is absolutely necessary for man's maintenance of strength and energy, and that such form of Prana is absorbed from the food by the nerves of the tongue, mouth and teeth. The act of mastication liberates this Prana, by separating the particles of the food into minute bits, thus exposing as many atoms of Prana to the tongue, mouth and teeth as possible. Each atom of food contains numerous electrons of food-prana, or food energy, which electrons are liberated by the breaking-up process of mastication, and the chemical action of certain subtle chemical constituents of the saliva, the presence of which have not been suspected by modern scientists, and which are not discernible by the tests of modern chemistry, although future investigators will scientifically prove their existence. Once liberated from the food, this food-prana flies to the nerves of the tongue, mouth and teeth, passing through the flesh and bone readily, and is rapidly conveyed to numerous storage-houses of the nervous system, from whence it is conveyed to all parts of the body, where it is used to furnish energy and "vitality" to the cells. This is a bare statement of the theory, the details of which we will endeavour to fill in as we proceed.

The student will probably wonder why it is necessary to extract this food-prana, as the air is heavily charged with Prana, and it may seem like a waste of effort on the part of Nature to use so much energy in order to extract the Prana from the food. But here is the explanation. Just as all electricity is electricity, so is all Prana simply Prana—but just as there are several forms of the electric current, manifesting widely different effects upon the human body, so are there several manifestations or forms of Prana, each of which performs certain work in the physical body, and all of which are needed for the different kinds of work. The Prana of the air fulfils certain offices; that of the water others, and that derived from the food still a third set of duties. To go into the minute details of the Yogi theory would be foreign to the purposes of this work, and we must rest content with the general statements here given. The main subject before us is the fact that the food contains food-prana, which the human body needs, and which it can extract only in the manner above stated, *i.e.*, by mastication of the food, and the absorption of the prana by the nervous system by means of the nerves of the tongue, mouth and teeth.

Now, let us consider Nature's plan in combining two important offices in the act of masticating and insalivating. In the first place, nature intended every particle of food to be thoroughly masticated and insalivated before it was swallowed, and any neglect in this respect is sure to be followed by imperfect digestion. Thorough mastication is a natural habit of man which has been neglected owing to the demands of artificial habits of living which have grown up around our civilization. Mastication is necessary to break up the food that it may be more easily swallowed, and also that it may be mixed with the saliva and the digestive juices of the stomach and small intestines. It promotes the flow of saliva, which is a most necessary part of the process of digestion. Insalivation of food is part of the digestive process, and certain work is done by the saliva which cannot be performed by the other digestive juices. Physiologists teach most positively that thorough mastication and proper insalivation of the food are pre-requisites of normal digestion, and form a most necessary part of the process. Certain specialists have gone much further and have given to the process of mastication and insalivation much more importance than have the general run of physiologists. One particular authority, Mr. Horace Fletcher, an American writer, has written most forcibly upon this subject, and has given startling proofs of the importance of this function and process of the physical body ; in fact, Mr. Fletcher advises a particular form of mastication which corresponds very closely to the Yogi custom, although he advises it because of its wonderful effect upon the digestion, whereas the Yogis practise a similar system upon the theory of the absorption of food-prana. The truth is that *both* results are accomplished, it being a part of Nature's strategy that the grinding of the food into small bits ; the digestive process attending the insalivation, and the absorption of food-prana, are accomplished at the same time—an economy of force most remarkable.

In the natural state of man, mastication was a most pleasant process, and so it is in the case of the lower animals, and the children of the human race to-day. The animal chews and munches his food with the greatest relish, and the child sucks, chews and holds in the mouth the food much longer than does the adult, until it begins to take lessons from its parents and acquires the custom of bolting its food. Mr. Fletcher, in his books on the subject, takes the position that it is taste which affords the pleasure of this chewing and sucking process. The Yogi theory is that while taste has much to do with it, still there is a something else, an indescribable sense of satisfaction obtained from holding the food in the mouth, rolling it around with the tongue, masticating it and allowing it to dissolve slowly and be swallowed almost unconsciously. Fletcher holds that while there remains a particle of taste in the food, nourishment is there to be extracted, and we believe this to be strictly correct. But we hold that there is that other sensation which, when we allow it to manifest itself, gives us a certain satisfaction in the non-swallowing, and which sensation continues until all, or nearly all, the food-prana is extracted from the food. You will notice if you follow the Yogi plan of eating (even partially) that you will be loth to part with the food, and that, instead of bolting it at once, you will allow it to gradually melt away in the mouth until suddenly you realize that it is all gone. And this sensation is experienced from the plainest kinds of food, which do not appeal particularly to the taste, as well as to those foods which are special favourites of your particular taste.

To describe this sensation is almost impossible, for we have no English words coined for it, as its existence has not been fully recognized by the Western races. The best we can do is to compare it by other sensations at the risk of being accused of presenting a ridiculous comparison or illustration. Here is what we mean : You know the sensation which one sometimes feels when in the presence of a highly " magnetic " person—that indescribable feeling of the absorption of strength or " vitality." Some people have so much Prana in their system that they are continually " running over " and giving it out to others, the result being that other persons like to be in their company, and dislike to leave it, being almost unable to tear themselves away. This is one instance. Another is the sensation which one obtains from being close to another whom one loves. In this case there is an interchange of " magnetism " (thought charged with Prana) which is quite exhilarating. A kiss from the loved one is so filled with " magnetism " that it thrills one from head to toe. This gives an imperfect illustration of what we are trying to describe. The pleasure that one obtains from proper and normal eating, is not alone a matter of taste, but is largely derived from that peculiar sensation of the absorption of "magnetism" or Prana, which is very much akin to the examples above mentioned, although, until one realizes the similar character of the two manifestations of energy, the illustration may evoke a smile, or possibly ridicule.

When one has overcome the false Appetite (so often mistaken for Hunger) he will masticate a dry crust of whole-wheat bread and not only obtain a certain satisfaction of taste from the nourishment contained within it, but will enjoy the sensation of which we have spoken very keenly. It takes a little practice in order to get rid of the false appetite habit and to return to Nature's plans. The most nourishing of foods will yield the most satisfaction to the normal taste, and it is a fact to be remembered that food-prana is contained in food in direct proportion to its percentage of nourishment—another instance of Nature's wisdom.

The Yogi eats his food slowly, masticating each mouthful so long as he "feels like it"; that is, so long as it yields him any satisfaction. In the majority of cases this sensation lasts so long as there remains any food in the mouth, as Nature's involuntary processes gradually causes the food to be slowly dissolved and swallowed. The Yogi moves his jaws slowly, and allows the tongue to caress the food, and the teeth to sink into it lovingly, knowing that he is extracting the food-prana from it, by means of the nerves of the mouth, tongue and teeth, and that he is being stimulated and strengthened, and that he is replenishing his reservoir of energy. At the same time he is conscious that he is preparing his food in the proper way for the digestive processes of the stomach and small intestines, and is giving his body good material needed for the building up of the physical body.

Those who follow the Yogi plan of eating will obtain a far greater amount of nourishment from their food than does the ordinary person, for every ounce is forced to yield up the maximum nourishment, while in the case of the man who bolts his food half-masticated and insufficiently insalivated, much goes to waste, and is passed from the system in the shape of a decaying, fermenting mass. Under the Yogi plan nothing is passed from the system as waste except the *real waste* matter, every particle of nourishment being extracted from the food, and the greater portion of the food-prana being absorbed from its atoms. The mastication breaks up the food into small particles, allowing the fluids of the saliva to interpenetrate it, the digestive juices of the saliva performing their necessary work, and the other juices (mentioned above) acting upon the atoms of food in such a way as to liberate the food-prana, thus allowing it to be taken up by the nervous system. The motion imparted to the food by the action of the jaws, tongue and cheeks in the act of mastication, causes it to present new atoms to the nerves ready to extract the food-prana. The Yogis hold the food in the mouth, masticating it slowly and thoroughly, and allowing it to be slowly swallowed by the involuntary process above alluded to, and they experience to the full the enjoyment attendant upon the extraction of Prana. You may get an idea of this by taking into the mouth some particle of food (when you have plenty of time for the experiment), and then slowly masticating it, allowing it to gradually melt away in the mouth, as you would a lump of sugar. You will be surprised to find how thoroughly this work of involuntary swallowing is performed—the food gradually yields up its food-prana and then melts slowly away and reaches the stomach. Take a crust of bread, for example, and masticate it thoroughly, with the idea of seeing how long it will last without being "swallowed." You will find that it will never be "swallowed" in the usual way, but will gradually disappear in the manner we have just mentioned, after being reduced to a pasty, creamy mass by degrees. And that little mouthful of bread will have yielded you about twice as much nourishment as a piece of equal size, eaten in the ordinary way, and about three times the amount of food-prana.

Another interesting example is had in the case of milk. Milk is a fluid, and, of course, needs no "breaking-up," as does solid food. Yet the fact remains (and is well established by careful experiments) that a quart of milk simply allowed to flow down the throat yields not over half the nourishment or food-prana that is derived from the same quantity of milk sipped slowly, and allowed to remain in the mouth a moment until it "melts away," the tongue being moved through it. The babe drawing the milk from the nipple of either the breast or the bottle, of course, does so by a sucking motion, which moves the tongue and cheeks, and produces a flow of fluid from the glands, which liberates the food-prana and has also a chemical digestive effect upon the milk itself, notwithstanding the fact that true saliva is not secreted in the young babe, and does not appear until the teeth show themselves.

We advise our students to experiment with themselves along the lines just pointed out. Choose an opportunity when you have plenty of time, then, masticating slowly, allow the food to gradually melt away, instead of making a deliberate attempt to swallow. This "melting-away" of the food can only be possible when the food is masticated into a cream-like paste, thoroughly saturated with saliva, and the particles thereby converted into a semi-digested state, and having had the food-prana extracted therefrom. Try eating an apple in this way, and you will be surprised at the feeling of having eaten a fair-sized meal, and at the sensation of increased strength which has come to you.

We understand fully that it is quite a different thing for the Yogi to take his time and eat in this way, and for the hurried Western man of business to do the same, and we do not expect all of our readers to change the habit of years all at once. But we feel sure that a little practice in this method of eating food will cause quite a change to come over one, and we know that such occasional practice will soon result in quite an improvement in the everyday method of masticating the food. We know, also, that the student will find a new delight—an additional relish in eating—and will soon learn to eat "lovingly," that is, to feel loth to let the mouthful of food pass away. A new world of taste is opened up to the man who learns to follow this plan, and he will get far more pleasure from eating than ever before, and will have, besides, a much better digestion, and much more vitality, for he will obtain a greater degree of nourishment, and an increased amount of food-prana.

It is possible for one who has the time and opportunity to follow this plan to its extreme limit, to obtain an almost unbelievable amount of nourishment and strength from a comparatively small amount of food, as there will be practically no waste, as may be proven by an observation of the waste matter which is passed from the system. Those suffering from malnutrition and impaired vitality will find it profitable to at least partially follow this plan.

The Yogis are known as small eaters, and yet they understand fully the necessity and value of perfect nutrition, and always keep the body well nourished and provided with building material. The secret, as you will readily see, is that they waste practically none of the nourishment in the food, as they extract practically all that it contains. They do not burden their system with waste material, which clogs up the machinery and causes a waste of energy in order that it may be thrown off. They obtain a maximum of nourishment from a minimum of food—a full supply of food-prana from a small amount of material.

While you may not be able to follow this matter up to the extreme, you may work a great improvement in yourself by following the methods above given. We merely give you the general principles—work the rest out for yourself—experiment for yourself—that is the only way to learn anything, anyway.

We have stated several times in this book, that the mental attitude aids materially in the process of absorbing Prana. This is true not only of the Prana absorbed from the air, but also of the food-prana. Hold the thought that you are absorbing all the Prana contained in a mouthful of food, combining that thought with that of " Nourishment," and you will be able to do much more than you can without so doing.

CHAPTER XI

ABOUT FOOD

We intend to leave the matter of the choice of food an open question with our students. While, personally, we prefer certain kinds of food, believing that the best results are obtained from the use thereof, we recognize the fact that it is impossible to change the habits of a lifetime (yes, of many generations) in a day, and man must be guided by his own experience and his growing knowledge, rather than by dogmatic utterances of others. The Yogis prefer a non-animal diet, both from hygienic reasons and the Oriental aversion to eating the flesh of animals. The more advanced of the Yogi students prefer a diet of fruit, nuts, olive oil, etc., together with a form of unleavened bread made from the entire wheat. But when they travel among those who follow different dietary rules from themselves they do not hesitate to adapt themselves to the changed conditions, to a greater or less extent, and do not render themselves a burden to their hosts, knowing that if they follow the Yogi plan of masticating their food slowly their stomachs will take good care of what they eat. In fact, some of the most indigestible things in the modern menu may be safely eaten if the above mentioned system is adopted.

And we write this chapter in the spirit of the travelling Yogi. We have no wish to force arbitrary rules upon our students. Man must grow into a more rational method of eating, rather than have it forced upon him suddenly. It is hard for one to adopt a non-meat diet, if he has been used to animal flesh all his life, and it is equally difficult for one to take up an uncooked dietary list, if he has been eating cooked dishes all his life. All we ask of you is to think a little on the subject and to trust your own instinct regarding the choice of food, giving yourself as great a variety as possible. The instinct, if trusted, will usually cause you to select that which you need for that particular meal, and we would prefer to trust the instinct rather than to bind ourselves to any fixed, unchangeable dietary. Eat pretty much what you feel like, providing you masticate it thoroughly and slowly, and give yourself a wide range of choice. We will speak, in this chapter, of a few things which the rational man will avoid but will do so merely in the way of general advice. In the matter of non-meat eating, we believe that mankind will gradually grow to feel that meat is not its proper diet, but we believe that one must outgrow that feeling, rather than to have it beaten out of him, for if he "longs" for the flesh-pots of Egypt, it is about as bad as if he really participated in the feast. Man will cease to desire meat, as he grows, but until that time comes, any forced restraint of the meat habit will not do him much good. We are aware that this will be considered heterodox by many of our readers, but we cannot help that fact—our statements will stand the test of experience.

If our students are interested in the question of the relative advantages of particular kinds of foods, let them read some of the very good works which have been written upon the subject of recent years. But let them read upon the several sides of the question, and avoid being carried away by the particular fad of the writer whose book is before them. It is instructive and interesting to read of the comparative food values of the various articles upon our tables, and such knowledge will gradually tend to a more rational dietary. But such changes must be the result of thought and experience, rather than upon the mere say so of some person riding a hobby. We suggest that our students consider whether or not they are eating too much meat; whether they are living upon too much fat and grease; whether they are eating enough fruit; whether whole-wheat bread would not be a good addition to their bill of fare; whether they are not indulging in too much pastry and "made dishes." If we were asked to give them a general rule regarding eating we would be apt to say, "Eat a variety of foods; avoid 'rich' dishes; do not eat too much fat; beware of the frying-pan; do not eat too much meat; avoid, especially, pig meat and veal; let your general habit of eating tend toward the simple, plain fare, rather than toward the elaborate dishes; go slow on pastry; cut out hot cakes from your list; masticate thoroughly and slowly, according to the plan we have given you; don't be afraid of food, if you eat it properly it will not hurt you, providing you do not fear it."

We think it better to make the first meal of the day a light one, as there is very little waste to repair in the morning, as the body has been at rest all night. If possible, take a little exercise before breakfast.

If you once return to the natural habit of proper mastication, and experience the sensation that comes from proper eating, the abnormal appetites which have been acquired will fall from you, and natural hunger will return. When natural hunger is with you, the instinct will be very keen in picking out nutritious food for you, and you will feel inclined toward that which will give you just the nourishment you need at any particular time. Man's instinct is a good guide, providing it has not been spoiled by the indulgence in the absurd dishes so common in these days, which create false appetite.

If you feel "out of sorts," do not be afraid to "cut out" a meal, and give the stomach a chance to get rid of what it has on hand. One can go without eating for a number of days without danger, although we do not advise prolonged fasts. We feel, however, that in sickness it is wise to give the stomach a rest, in order that the recuperative energy may be directed toward the casting out of the waste matter which has been causing the trouble. You will notice that the animals stop eating while they are sick, and lie around until health is restored, when they return to their meals. We may take this lesson from them with considerable profit.

We do not wish students to become "food cranks" who weigh, measure and analyze every mouthful of food. We consider this an abnormal method and believe that such a course generates fear-thought and fills the Instinctive mind with all sorts of erroneous ideas. We think it a much better plan to use ordinary precautions and judgment in the selection of one's food, and then to bother no more about the matter, but eat with the thought of nourishment and strength in your minds, masticating the food as we have stated, and knowing that nature will do its work well. Keep as close to nature as possible, and let her plans be your standard of measurement. The strong, healthy man is not afraid of his food, and neither should be the man who wishes to be healthy. Keep cheerful, breathe properly, eat properly, live properly, and you will not have occasion to make a chemical analysis of every mouthful of food. Do not be afraid to trust to your instinct, for that is the natural man's guide, after all.

CHAPTER XII

THE IRRIGATION OF THE BODY

ONE of the cardinal principles of the Hatha Yoga Philosophy of Health is the intelligent use of Nature's great gift to living things—Water. It should not be necessary to even call the attention of men to the fact that Water is one of the great means of maintaining normal health, but man has become so much a slave to artificial environments, habits, customs, etc., that he has forgotten Nature's laws. His only hope is to return to Nature. The little child knows, instinctively, the use of water, and insists upon being furnished with it, but as it grows older it gets away from the natural habit, and falls into the erroneous practices of the older people around it. This is particularly true of those living in large cities, where they find unpalatable the warm water drawn from faucets, and so gradually become weaned away from the normal use of fluids. Such persons gradually form new habits of drinking (or not drinking), and, putting off Nature's demands, they at last are not conscious of them. We often hear people say, " But why should we drink water—we do not get thirsty? " But had they continued in Nature's paths they *would* get thirsty, and the only reason why they do not hear Nature's calls is because they have so long turned a deaf ear to her that she has become discouraged and cries less loudly; besides, their ears have ceased to recognize the vibrations, being so much taken up with other things. It is astonishing to find how people neglect this important feature of life. Many drink scarcely any fluids, and even say that they do not think it is "good for them." This has gone so far that we know of one so called "health teacher" who puts forth the astounding theory that "Thirst is a Disease," and counsels people against the use of fluids at all, stating that the use of them is unnatural. We will not attempt to argue with such teachings—their folly must be apparent to anyone who will look at the natural life habits of man and the lower animals. Let man go back to Nature, and he will see water-drinking all around him, in all forms of life, from the plant up to the highest mammal.

So much importance does the Yogi attach to the proper use of drinking water, that he considers it one of the first principles of health. He knows that a large percentage of sick people are sick because of their lack of the fluids which the body requires. Just as the plant needs water, as well as the food derived from the soil and air, to bring it to healthy maturity, so does man require the proper amount of fluids to keep him in health, or to bring him again to health in case he has lost it. Who would think of depriving a plant of water? And who would be so cruel as to fail to provide the faithful horse with the requisite amount of water? And yet, man, while giving the plant and the animal that which his common sense teaches him they require, will deprive himself of the life-giving fluid, and will suffer the consequences, just as would the plant and horse under similar conditions. Keep this example of plant and horse before you when you consider the question of drinking water.

Let us see what water is used for in the body, and then make up our minds whether or not we have been living normal lives in this respect.

In the first place, about 70 per cent. of our physical body is water ! A certain amount of this water is being used up by our system, and leaves the body constantly, and every ounce that is used up must be replaced by another ounce if the body is to be kept in a normal condition.

The system is continuously excreting water through the pores of the skin, in the shape of sweat and perspiration. Sweat is the term applied to such excretion when it is thrown off so rapidly that it gathers and collects in drops. Perspiration is the term applied when the water is continuously and unconsciously evaporated from the skin. Perspiration is continuously being evaporated from the skin, and experiments have shown that when it is prevented the animal dies. In one of the festivals of ancient Rome a boy was covered with gold-leaf, from head to foot, in order to represent one of the gods—he died before the gold-leaf could be removed, the perspiration being unable to penetrate the varnish and the leaf. Nature's function was interrupted and the body being unable to function properly, the soul threw off its fleshly tenement.

Sweat and perspiration are shown by chemical analysis to be loaded with the waste products of the system—the refuse and filth of the body—which, without a sufficient supply of fluids in the system, would remain in the body, poisoning it and bringing disease and death as a consequence. The repair work of the body is continually going on, the used-up and worn-out tissue being carried off and replaced by fresh, new material from the blood, which has absorbed it from the nutrition in the food. This waste must be cast out of the body, and Nature is quite particular that it shall be gotten rid of—she does not favour the storing up of garbage in the system. If this waste matter is allowed to remain in the system it becomes a poison and breeds diseased conditions—it serves as a breeding place and a feeding ground for germs, microbes, spores and bacteria, and all the rest of that family. Germs do not bother the clean and healthy system to any great extent, but let them come around one of these water-haters, and it finds his or her body full of uncast-off refuse and filth, and they settle down to business. We will have something more to say along this line when we come to the subject of Bathing.

Water plays a most important part in the every-day life of the Hatha Yogi. He uses it internally and externally. He uses it to keep healthy, and he teaches its value to bring about healthy conditions, where disease has impaired the natural functioning of the body. We will touch upon the use of water in several parts of this book. We wish to impress upon our students the importance of the subject, begging them not to pass it by as unimportant because it is so simple. Seven out of ten of our readers need this advice. Do not pass it by. THIS MEANS YOU.

Both perspiration and sweat are necessary, also,

to dissipate the excessive bodily heat by their evaporation, and thus keep down the bodily temperature to a normal degree. The perspiration and sweat also (as we have stated) assist in carrying off the waste products of the system—the skin being, in fact, a supplementary organ to the kidneys. And without water the skin would, of course, be unable to perform this function.

The normal adult excretes about one and one-half to two pints of water in twenty-four hours, in the shape of sweat and perspiration, but men working in rolling-mills, etc., excrete much greater quantities. One can endure a much greater degree of heat in a dry atmosphere than in a moist one, because in the former the perspiration is evaporated so rapidly that the heat is more readily and rapidly dissipated.

Quite a quantity of water is exhaled through the lungs. The urinary organs pass off a large quantity, in performing their functions, about three pints in twenty-four hours being the amount voided by the normal adult. And all this has to be replenished, in order to keep the physical machinery going right.

Water is needed by the system for a number of purposes. One of its purposes (as above stated) is to counteract and regulate the combustion constantly going on in our bodies, arising from the chemical action of the oxygen extracted by the lungs from the air, coming in contact with the carbon arising from the food. This combustion going on in millions of cells produces the animal heat. The water passing through the system regulates this combustion, so that it does not become too intense.

Water is also used by the body as a common

carrier. It flows through the arteries and veins, and conveys the blood corpuscles and elements of nutrition to the various parts of the body, that they may be used in the building up process, which we have described. Without fluids in the system, the quantity of blood must decrease. On the return trip of the blood through the veins, the fluids take up the waste matter (much of which would be a rank poison if allowed to remain in the system), and carries it to the excretory organism of the kidneys, the pores of the skin, and lungs, where the poisonous dead material and waste of the system is thrown off. Without sufficient fluids this work cannot be accomplished as Nature intended. And (this a most important matter) without sufficient water the waste portions of the food—the ashes of the system—cannot be kept sufficiently moist to easily pass through the colon and out of the body, and Constipation, with all of its attendant evils, results. The Yogis know that nine-tenths of the cases of chronic constipation arise from this cause—they also know that nine-tenths of the cases of chronic constipation may be speedily cured by the returning to the natural habit of drinking water. We will devote a special chapter to this subject, but we wish to direct the attention of the reader to its importance, as often as possible.

Yes, a sufficient supply of water is needed to aid in the proper stimulation and circulation of the blood—in the elimination of the waste products of the system—and in the normal assimilation of nourishment by the system.

Persons who do not drink sufficient fluids almost

invariably are deficient in their supply of blood—they are often bloodless-looking creatures—pale, sallow, bloodless-looking anaemic creatures. Their skin is often dry and feverish, and they perspire but little. They have an unhealthy appearance, and remind one of dried fruit, needing a good soaking to make them look plump and normal. They are nearly always sufferers from constipation—and constipation brings with it a myriad of other disorders, as we will show you in another chapter. Their large intestines, or colon, are unclean, and the system is continually absorbing the products of the waste stored away there, and endeavouring to get rid of it by means of foul breath; strong, sweaty perspiration, and unnatural urine. This is not pleasant reading, but it is necessary to use plain words when calling your attention to these things. And all this for the lack of a little water—just think of it. You who are so particular to keep yourselves clean on the outside, allow yourselves to remain filthy within.

Man's body needs water all over its inner parts. It needs constant irrigation, and if that irrigation is denied the bodies suffer just as does the land, denied its natural supply of water. Every cell, tissue and organ needs water in order to be healthy. Water is a universal solvent and enables the system to assimilate and distribute the nourishment obtained from the food, and to get rid of the waste products of the system. It is often said that the "blood is the life," and if this is so, what must the water be called—for without water the blood would be but dust?

Water is needed also for the purpose of enabling the kidneys to perform their functions of carrying off the urea, etc. It is needed in order to be manufactured into saliva, bile, pancreatic juice, gastric juices, and all the other valuable juices of the system, without which digestion would be impossible. Shut off your supply of fluids, and you decrease your supply of all of these necessary things. Do you realize that?

If you doubt these facts, thinking them to be but theories of the Yogis, you have but to refer to any good scientific work upon physiology, written by any of the Western authorities upon the subject. You will find all that we have told you fully corroborated there. A well-known Western physiologist has said that so much water exists in the tissues of a normal system that it may be asserted as an axiom that "all organisms live in water." And if there is no water, there can be no life, or health.

You have been shown that the kidneys secrete about three pints of urine in twenty-four hours, which is passed off from the system, carrying in solution waste products and poisonous chemical substances which have been gathered up from the system by the kidneys. In addition to this, we have shown you that the skin excretes from one and one-half pints to two pints of water, in the shape of sweat and perspiration, in the same time. In addition to this there is a moderate quantity (average ten to fifteen ounces) given off by the lungs in exhalation during the same time. Besides a certain amount passes off through the excretions from the bowels. And a small amount is passed from the system in the shape of tears, and other secretions and excretions of the body. Now, how much water is needed to renew this waste? Let us see. A certain amount of fluids is taken into the system with the food, particularly when certain kinds of food are eaten. But this is only a comparatively small portion of what has been thrown off from the system in its cleansing functions. The best authorities agree that from two quarts to five pints of water is the amount necessary to be taken daily by the average, normal man and woman, in order to make up the waste. If that amount is not supplied to the body it will withdraw fluids from the system until the person assumes that "dried-up" state of which we have spoken, with the consequence that all the physical functions are impaired, the persons being "dried-up" inside as well as on the surface—the machinery of the body being deprived of its lubricating and cleansing material.

Two quarts a day! Just think of that, you people who have been taking about one pint, or even less, each day! Do you wonder why you are afflicted with all sorts of bodily ailments? No wonder you are dyspeptic, constipated, bloodless, nervous and generally all out of sorts. Your bodies are filled with all sorts of poisonous substances which Nature has not been able to eliminate and throw off through the kidneys and skin, because you have shut off her water supply. No wonder your colons are filled with impacted waste matter, which is poisoning your system, and which Nature has been unable to pass off in the regular way because you did not give her water with which to flush her sewers. No wonder that your saliva and gastric juices are deficient—how do you suppose Nature can manufacture them without sufficient water? No wonder your blood is deficient in quantity—where do you suppose Nature is going to get the fluids from to make the blood? No wonder that your nerves are our of condition, with all this abnormal going on. Poor Nature does the best she can, even though you be foolish. She draws a little water from the system in order that the machinery shall not entirely stop, but she dare not draw too much—so she compromises. She does just as you do when the water in the spring is nearly exhausted—you try to make a little do the work of much, and must rest content with doing things only half-way right.

The Yogis are not afraid to drink a sufficient amount of water each day. They are not afraid of "thinning the blood," as are some of these "dried-up" people. Nature throws off the surplus quantity if it be taken, very readily and rapidly. They do not crave "ice water"—an unnatural product of civilization(?)—their favourite temperature is about 60 degrees. They drink when they are thirsty—and they have a normal thirst which does not have to be restored as does that of the "dried-up" people. They drink frequently, but mark ye this: *they do not drink large quantities at any one time.* They do not "pour the water down," believing that such a practice is abnormal and unnatural, and injurious. They drink it in small quantities, though often during the day. When working they often keep a vessel of water near them, and frequently sip therefrom.

Those who have neglected their natural instincts for many years have almost forgotten the natural habit of water drinking, and need considerable practice to regain it. A little practice will soon begin to create a demand for water, and you will in time regain the natural thirst. A good plan is to keep a glass of water near you, and take an occasional sip from it, thinking at the same time what you are taking it for. Say to yourself: "I am giving my body the fluids it requires to do its work properly, and it will respond by bringing normal conditions back to me—giving me good health and strength, and making me a strong, healthy, natural man (or woman)."

The Yogis drink a cupful of water the last thing before going to bed at night. This is taken up by the system and is used in cleansing the body during the night, the waste products being excreted with the urine in the morning. They also drink a cupful immediately after arising in the morning, the theory being that by taking the water before eating it cleanses the stomach and washes away the sediment and waste which have settled during the night. They usually drink a cupful about an hour before each meal, following it by some mild exercise, believing that this prepares the digestive apparatus for the meal, and promotes natural hunger. They are not afraid of drinking a little water even at meals (imagine the horror of some of our "health-teachers" when they read this), but are careful not to "wash down" their food with water. Washing down the food with water not only dilutes the saliva, but causes one to swallow his food imperfectly insalivated and masticated—makes it go down before Nature is ready—and interferes with the Yogi method of masticating the food (see chapter on same). The

Yogis believe that only in this way is water harmful when taken at meals—and for the reason given, alone—they take a little at each meal to soften up the food mass in the stomach, and that little does not weaken the strength of the gastric-juices, etc.

Many of our readers are familiar with the use of hot water as a means of cleansing a foul stomach. We approve of its use in that way, when needed, but we think that if our students will carefully follow the Yogi plan of living, as given in this book, they will have no foul stomachs needing cleansing—their stomachs will be good, healthy ones. As a preliminary toward rational eating, the sufferer may find it advantageous to use hot water in this way. The best way is to take about one pint, slowly sipping it, in the morning before breakfast, or about one hour before other meals. It will excite a muscular action in the digestive organs, which will tend to pass from the system the foul matter stored up there, which the hot water has loosened up and diluted, as well. But this is only a temporary expedient. Nature did not contemplate hot water as steady beverage, and water at ordinary temperature is all that she requires in health—and that she requires to maintain health—but when health has been lost through disobedience to her laws, hot water is a good thing with which to clean house before resuming natural habits.

We will have more to say about the use of water in Bathing, outward application, etc., in other parts of this book—this chapter is devoted to its internal offices.

In addition to the properties, offices and uses of water, as above given, we will add that water contains Prana in considerable quantities, a portion of which it parts with in the system, particularly if the system demands it and extracts it. One often feels the need of a cupful of water as a stimulant—the reason being that for some reason the normal supply of Prana has become depleted—and Nature, recognizing that it may obtain Prana rapidly and easily from water, causes the demand. You all remember how at times a cup of cool water has acted as a powerful stimulant and "refresher" to you, and how it enabled you to return to your work with renewed vigour and energy. Do not forget Water when you feel "used up." Used in connection with Yogi Breathing it will give a man fresh energy quicker than will any other method.

In sipping water, let it remain in the mouth a moment before swallowing. The nerves of the tongue and mouth are the first (and quickest) to absorb the Prana, and this plan will prove advantageous, particularly when one is tired. This is worth remembering

CHAPTER XIII

THE ASHES OF THE SYSTEM

THIS will not be a pleasant chapter to those of you who are still bound with the old notions of the impurity of the body, or any part of it—if there chance to be such among our students. Those of you who prefer to ignore the existence of certain important functions of the physical body, and feel a sense of shame at the thought that certain physical functions are a part of their everyday lives, will not relish this chapter, and may even regard it as a blot upon the book—a thing which we should have omitted—something which we should have ignored. To such we would say that we can see no use (and much harm) in following the policy of the ostrich in the old tale, who, dreading his hunters, would stick his head in the sand, and, shutting the hated things from sight, would ignore their existence until they overtook and captured him. We have such respect for the entire human body, and all its parts and functions, that we are unable to see anything impure or " un-nice " about it. And we can see nothing but folly in the policy which refuses to consider and discuss the functions referred to, or any others. The result of this conventional policy of dodging the unpleasant subjects, has been that many of the race are suffering from diseases and ill health brought about by this folly. To many who read this chapter, what we say will come as a new revelation—others who are already acquainted with that of which we speak, will welcome the voicing of the truth in this book, knowing that many will be benefited by having their attention called to it. We purpose giving you a plain talk about the ashes of the system—the cast-off waste of the body.

That such a talk is needed, is evidenced by the fact that at least three-quarters of the modern people are sufferers from a greater or lesser degree of constipation and its baneful results. This is all contrary to nature, and the cause is so easily removed that one can scarcely imagine why this state of affairs is allowed to continue. There can be but one answer—ignorance of the cause and cure. If we are able to aid in the work of removing this curse of the race, and in thus restoring normal conditions by bringing people back to nature, we will not mind the disgusted expression upon the faces of some who glance at this chapter and turn to some more pleasant subject—these very people being the ones who need this advice the most of any of our readers.

Those who have read the chapter in this book upon the Digestive Organs, will remember that we left the subject at the stage where the food was in the small intestines, being absorbed and taken up by the system. Our next point is to consider what becomes of the waste products of the food after the system has taken up all the nourishment it can from it—the material which it cannot use.

Right here it will be as well to state that those who follow the Yogi plan of eating their food, as given in other chapters, will have a much less amount of this waste matter than the average man or woman who allows his or her food to reach the stomach only partially prepared for digestion and assimilation. The average person wastes at least half of what he eats—the waste matter of those who follow the Yogi practice being comparatively small and much less offensive than that of the average person.

In order to understand our subject, we must take a look at the organs of the body having to do with it. The large intestine of the "Colon" (the large bowel) is the part of the body to be considered. The colon is a large canal nearly five feet in length, passing up from the lower right-hand side of the abdomen, then passing over to the upper left-hand side, then passing down again to the lower left-hand side, where it makes sort of a twist or curve, and grows smaller, terminating in the rectum or exit of the waste matter of the system.

The small intestine empties into the colon by means of a small trap-door arrangement, on the lower right-hand side of the abdomen; this trap-door is so arranged that it allows matter to pass out, but will not allow it to pass back. The Vermiform Appendix, the seat of appendicitis, is just below this entrance. The colon rises straight up on the right-hand side of the abdomen, then makes a curve and passes right over to the upper left-hand side; then descends straight to the lower left-hand side, where the peculiar twist or curve called the Sigmoid Flexure occurs, following which is the rectum or smaller canal leading to the anus, which is the opening in the body through which the waste matter passes out of the body.

The colon is a great big sewer through which should pass freely the sewerage of the system. Nature intends this sewage to be removed speedily, and man in his natural state, like the animals, does not long delay this necessary casting off. But as he grows more civilized, he does not find it so convenient, and so he postpones nature's calls, until at last she gets tired of calling his attention to the matter, and goes off and attends to some of her other numerous duties. Man helps along this abnormal unnatural state of affairs by neglecting to partake of sufficient water, and not only does not give the colon sufficient fluids to properly moisten, soften and loosen the waste matter on its way from the system, but he even lets his body run so short of fluids that nature, in desperation, draws back through the walls of the colon some of the water already given it for its use—failing to get spring water for her work, she must needs use sewer water. Imagine the result! The failure of man to allow a free passage of this refuse matter from the colon results in constipation, which is the source of innumerable cases of ill health, the real nature of which is generally not suspected. Many people who have a movement of the bowels each day are really constipated, although they do not know it. The walls of the colon are encrusted with impacted waste matter, some of which has been there for many days, a small opening in the middle of the mass allowing what is absolutely necessary to pass through. Constipation means a state in which the colon is not perfectly clean and free of impacted faecal matter.

A colon filled, or partially filled, with old faecal

matter is a source of poison to the whole system. The colon has walls which absorb the contents of the colon. Medical practice demonstrates that nourishment injected into the colon will be absorbed rapidly and carried to the blood. Drugs injected in the same way reach the other parts of the system. And as before stated, the fluid portion of the waste faecal matter is absorbed by the system, the sewage water being used in nature's work because of the shortage of purer fluids in the system. It is almost incredible how long old faecal matter will remain in a constipated colon. Cases are on record showing that when the colon is cleaned, among the masses of old faecal matter has been found cherry stones, etc., eaten several months before. Cathartics do not remove this old faecal matter, as they simply loosen up what is in the stomach and small intestines, and pass it off through the little opening in the hardened faecal matter with which the walls of a badly constipated colon is lined. In some persons the colon is impacted with hardened faeces, almost as solid as soft coal, to such an extent that their abdomens become swollen and hard. This old waste matter becomes sometimes so foul that it becomes the breeding place of worms, and even maggots, and the colon is filled with their eggs. The waste matter, or faeces, which is passed into the colon from the small intestine, is of a pasty substance, and if the bowels are clear and clean, and the movements natural, it should pass from the system in but a trifle more solid state, and of a light colour. The longer faecal matter is retained in the colon, the harder and drier it becomes, and the darker in colour. When sufficient fluids are not taken, and nature's calls are ignored until a more convenient time, and then forgotten, a drying up and hardening process ensues. When later the movement is had, only a portion of the faeces passes out, the balance remaining to clog up the colon. Next day a little more is added, and so on, until a case of chronic constipation is manifested, with all its attendant evils, such as dyspepsia, biliousness, liver troubles, kidney troubles—in fact, all diseases are encouraged, and many of them directly caused by this filthy condition of the colon. Half of the cases of female trouble are caused or aggravated by this condition.

The absorption by the blood of the faecal matter in the system, is occasioned in two ways, first, the desire and need of the body for fluids; second, a desperate effort of nature to throw off the waste matter by the skin, the kidneys and the lungs. Foul perspiration and foul breath are often caused by this effort of nature to get rid of what should have passed from the colon. Nature recognizes the great source of danger of allowing this foul mass to stay in the system, and so resorts to the desperate plan of throwing it off in other ways, even at the risk of half-poisoning the blood and body in so doing. The best proof of the number of physical ailments and disease caused by this unnatural state of the colon, is the fact that when the cause is once removed people begin to recover from many ailments apparently unconnected with the cause. In addition to the fact that diseases are caused and encouraged by this state of the colon, it is a fact that one is far more likely to contract contagious diseases, and diseases like typhoid fever, etc., by reason of a neglected colon furnishing a fine breeding place for the germs of these diseases. In fact a man who keeps his colon clean and healthy, is believed to run but very little risk of diseases of this kind. Just imagine what must be the result when we carry a sewer around inside of us—is it any wonder that diseases which are occasioned by filthy conditions outside thrive on like condition inside of the body? Use a little reason, friends.

Now that we have said enough to call your attention to the seat of many troubles (we could fill hundreds of pages with still stronger remarks on this subject) you are perhaps in a condition to ask: "Well, I believe that all this is true, and that it explains much that has been troubling me, but what must I do to get rid of that foul condition, and to regain and keep normal health in this respect?" Well, our answer is: "First get rid of the abnormal filthy accumulation, and then keep yourself sweet and clean and healthy, by following nature's laws. We will endeavour to show you how to do both of these things."

If the colon is but slightly filled with impacted faeces, one may get rid of it by increasing the fluids and by encouraging regular movements, and by treating the intelligence of the cells of the stomach (as hereinafter described). But, as over half of the people who are mentally asking us this question, have colons more or less filled with old, hardened, impacted faecal matter, of an almost green colour, which has been there for months, perhaps longer, we must give them a more radical remedy. As they have gone away from nature in contracting this trouble, we must aid nature somewhat in restoring lost conditions so that she may thereafter have a clean colon to work with. We will go to the animal kingdom for a suggestion. Many centuries ago the natives of India noticed that certain birds of the Ibis family—a long-billed bird—would return from journeys into the interior in a wretched condition, which was due either to their eating some berry which was very constipating, or else having been where there was no water to drink—possibly both. This bird would reach the rivers in an almost exhausted condition, scarcely able to fly from weakness. The bird would fill its bill and mouth with water from the river and then, inserting the bill into the rectum, would inject the water into the bowel, which would relieve it in a few moments. The bird would repeat this several times, until the bowel was completely emptied, and would then sit around and rest for a few minutes until its vitality was restored, when, after drinking freely from the river, it would fly away as strong and active as ever.

The chiefs and priests of the tribes noticing this occurrence, and its wonderful effect upon the birds, began to reason about the matter, and finally someone suggested that it might be tried to advantage upon some of the old men who, by reason of their non-activity and sedentary habits, had departed from nature's normal plan and had become constipated. So they managed to construct a primitive implement resembling a syringe from the reeds, with a sort of blow-pipe attachment, and would inject warm river water into the bowels of the old men suffering from this complaint. The results were wonderful—the old men took on a new lease of life, took unto themselves young wives, and began to again enter into the active work of the tribe, and to resume their positions as heads of the tribe, much to the amazement of the younger men who had considered the veterans out of the contest. The old men of other tribes heard of the occurrence and began coming in, borne on the shoulders of the young men—they are said to have walked home unaided. From all the accounts handed down, these primitive injections must have been of a most heroic character, for they speak of the use of "gallons of water," and by the time the treatment was concluded the colon of the old tribesmen must have been thoroughly cleaned out, and in a condition which would give the system no more poisons. But we are not going to advocate such heroic treatment—we are not tribesmen, remember.

Yes, the abnormal condition calls for a temporary aid to nature in getting rid of this foul accumulation in the colon. And the best way to get rid of it once and for all is to follow the example of the Ibis and the old Hindu tribesmen with the aid of perfected twentieth century apparatus. All that is needed is an ordinary cheap rubber syringe. If you have a fountain syringe, so much the better, but a cheap bulb syringe will do the work. Take a pint of pretty warm water—as warm as the hand can bear with comfort. Inject the water into the bowel with the syringe. Then hold the water in the colon for a few minutes, and then let it pass from the system. The night time is the best for this practice. The next night take a *quart* of warm water and use it the same way. Then skip a night, and the second night after, try three pints; then skip two nights, and the third night after try two quarts. You will gradually get used to retaining this quantity of water in the colon, and the larger amount will pretty well clean out the old matter, the smaller injections washing away the looser fragments, and generally dislodging and breaking up the hardened mass. Do not be afraid of the two quarts. Your colon will hold much more, and some persons use gallon injections, but we consider this rather too much. Knead the abdomen before and after the injection, and practice the Yogi Complete Breath after you get through, in order to stimulate you and generally equalize the circulation.

The result of these injections will not appeal to the æsthetic tastes of people, but the question is to get rid of the filth once and for all. The contents of the colon brought away by these initial injections are often of a most offensive and unpleasant nature, but certainly it is much better to have this filth out of your system than in it—it is just as foul when in you as when it is expelled. We have known of cases in which great lumps of faecal matter, hard and green as corroded copper, passed from people, and the stench arising from the vessel was such as to bring a most convincing proof of what harm had been wrought upon the system by its retention. No, this is not pleasant reading, but it is necessary in order to make you realize the importance of this internal cleaning. You will find that during the week in which you are cleansing the colon, you will have little or no natural movements of the bowels. Do not let this worry you, for it is caused by the water washing away that which ordinarily would have been evacuated in the stool. In a couple of days after the cleansing process is completed, you will begin to get down to natural and normal movements.

Now, right here, we wish to call your attention to the fact that we are not advocating the continuous use of the syringe—we do not consider it a natural habit, and fail to see its necessity, as we believe that natural habits persisted in will cause anyone to regain the normal movement of the bowels, without the use of any outside help. We advocate the syringe only as a preliminary measure in order to clear away past accumulations. We see no harm, however, in the use of the syringe, say once a month, as a preventative of a recurrence of the old conditions. There are several schools of teachers in America who advocate the use of the syringe as a daily duty. We cannot agree with them, for our motto is, "Get back to nature," and we believe that nature does not call for the daily use of the syringe. The Yogis believe that plenty of pure, fresh water, and a regular habit of going to stool, and a little "talking up" to the bowels, will do all that is necessary to keep one free from constipation.

After you are through with the week of syringe treatment (and even before that), start the normal use of drinking water, as we have explained in our chapter on that subject. Get the two quarts of fluids inside of you each day, and you will find quite an improvement. Then start the habit of going to the stool at the same time each day, whether you feel an inclination or not. You will gradually establish the habit, and nature is fond of falling into habits. Then again, you may really need an evacuation and not be aware of it, for you have deadened your nerve calls by repeated refusals to heed them, and you will have to begin all over again. Don't neglect this—it is simple but effective.

You will find it advantageous to give yourself auto-suggestions while sipping your cupful of water. Say to yourself, " I am drinking this water in order to supply my system with the fluids it needs. It will make my bowels move freely and regularly, as nature intended." Carry the idea in your mind of what you are trying to accomplish, and you will be apt to get your results quicker.

Now for an idea which may seem absurd to you, unless you understand the philosophy back of it. (We will tell you how to do it now, and talk about the philosophy in another chapter.) This consists in " talking up " to the bowel. Give the abdomen (along the lines of the colon) several gentle slaps with the hand, and say to it (yes, talk to it) : " Here, you Colon, I've given you a good cleaning out, and made you fresh and clean—I am giving you all the fluids you need to do your work properly—I am cultivating a regular habit in order to give you a chance to do your work—and now you've *got* to do it." Slap the region of the colon several times, saying, " And now you've *got* to do it." And you will find that the colon *will* do it. This seems like child's play to you, probably—you will understand the sense of it when you read the chapter on Involuntary Control. It is merely a simple way of accomplishing a scientific fact—a plain way of calling into play a mighty force.

Now, friends, if you have suffered from constipation,—and who has not?—you will find the above advice valuable. It will bring back those rosy cheeks and beautiful skin—it will banish that sallowness, that furred tongue, that foul breath, that troublesome liver, and all the rest of the family of symptoms arising from the clogged colon—that stopped up sewer which has been poisoning the body. Try this plan and you will begin to enjoy life, and to be a natural, clean, healthy being. And now in closing, fill up your glass with sparkling, clear, cool water, and join us in the toast, "Here's to health, and lots of it," and while you drink it down slowly, say to yourself, "This water is to bring me health and strength—it is Nature's own tonic."

CHAPTER XIV

YOGI BREATHING

LIFE is absolutely dependent upon the act of breathing. "Breath is Life."

Differ as they may upon details of theory and terminology, the Oriental and the Occidental agree upon these fundamental principles.

To breathe is to live, and without breath there is no life. Not only are the higher animals dependent upon breath for life and health, but even the lower forms of animal life must breathe to live, and plant life is likewise dependent upon the air for continued existence.

The infant draws in a long, deep breath, retains it for a moment to extract from it its life-giving properties, and then exhales it in a long wail, and lo! its life upon earth has begun. The old man gives a faint gasp, ceases to breathe, and life is over. From the first faint breath of the infant to the last gasp of the dying man, it is one long story of continued breathing. Life is but a series of breaths.

Breathing may be considered the most important of all of the functions of the body, for, indeed, all the other functions depend upon it. Man may exist some time without eating; a shorter time without drinking; but without breathing his existence may be measured by a few minutes.

And not only is Man dependent upon Breath for

life, but he is largely dependent upon correct habits of breathing for continued vitality and freedom from disease. An intelligent control of our breathing power will lengthen our days upon earth by giving us increased vitality and powers of resistance, and, on the other hand, unintelligent and careless breathing will tend to shorten our days, by decreasing our vitality and laying us open to disease.

Man in his normal state had no need of instruction in breathing. Like the lower animal and the child, he breathed naturally and properly, as nature intended him to do, but civilization has changed him in this and other respects. He has contracted improper methods and attitudes of walking, standing, and sitting, which have robbed him of his birthright of natural and correct breathing. He has paid a high price for civilization. The savage, to-day, breathes naturally, unless he has been contaminated by the habits of civilized man.

The percentage of civilized men who breathe correctly is quite small, and the result is shown in contracted chests, and stooping shoulders, and the terrible increase in diseases of the respiratory organs, including that dread monster, Consumption, "the white scourge." Eminent authorities have stated that one generation of correct breathers would regenerate the race, and disease would be so rare as to be looked upon as a curiosity. Whether looked at from the standpoint of the Oriental or Occidental, the connection between correct breathing and health is readily seen and explained.

The Occidental teachings show that the physical health depends very materially upon correct breathing. The Oriental teachers not only admit that their Occidental brothers are right, but say that in addition to the physical benefit derived from correct habits of breathing, man's mental power, happiness, self-control, clear-sightedness, morals, and even his spiritual growth may be increased by an understanding of the "Science of Breath." Whole schools of Oriental Philosophy have been founded upon this science, and this knowledge when grasped by the Western races, and by them put to the practical use which is their strong point, will work wonders among them. The theory of the East, wedded to the practice of the West, will produce worthy offspring.

This work will take up the Yogi "Science of Breath," which includes not only all that is known to the Western physiologists and hygienists, but the occult side of the subject as well. It not only points out the way to physical health along the lines of what Western scientists have termed "deep breathing," etc., but also goes into the less known phases of the subject.

The Yogi practises exercises by which he attains control of his body, and is enabled to send to any organ or part an increased flow of vital force or "prana," thereby strengthening and invigorating the part or organ. He knows all that his Western scientific brother knows about the physiological effect of correct breathing, but he also knows that the air contains more than oxygen and hydrogen and nitrogen, and that something more is accomplished than the mere oxygenating of the blood. He knows something about "prana," of which his

Western brother is ignorant, and he is fully aware of the nature and manner of handling that great principle of energy, and is fully informed as to its effect upon the human body and mind. He knows that by rhythmical breathing one may bring himself into harmonious vibration with nature, and aid in the unfoldment of his latent powers. He knows that by controlled breathing he may not only cure disease in himself and others, but also practically do away with fear and worry and the baser emotions.

In the consideration of the question of respiration, we must begin by considering the mechanical arrangements whereby the respiratory movements are effected. The mechanics of respiration manifest through (1) the elastic movements of the lungs, and (2) the activities of the sides and bottom of the thoracic cavity in which the lungs are contained. The thorax is that portion of the trunk between the neck and the abdomen, the cavity of which (known as the thoracic cavity) is occupied mainly by the lungs and heart. It is bounded by the spinal column, the ribs with their cartilages, the breastbone, and below by the diaphragm. It is generally spoken of as "the chest." It has been compared to a completely shut, conical box, the small end of which is turned upward, the back of the box being formed by the spinal column, the front by the breastbone and the sides by the ribs.

The ribs are twenty-four in number, twelve on each side, and emerge from each side of the spinal column. The upper seven pairs are known as "true ribs," being fastened to the breastbone direct, while the lower five pairs are called "false ribs" or "floating ribs," because they are not so fastened, the upper two of them being fastened by cartilage to the other ribs, the remainder having no cartilages, their forward ends being free.

The ribs are moved in respiration by two superficial muscular layers, known as the intercostal muscles. The diaphragm, the muscular partition before alluded to, separates the chest box from the abdominal cavity.

In the act of inhalation the muscles expand the lungs so that a vacuum is created and the air rushes in in accordance with the well known law of physics. Everything depends upon the muscles concerned in the process of respiration, which we may, for convenience, term the "respiratory muscles." Without the aid of these muscles the lungs cannot expand, and upon the proper use and control of these muscles the Science of Breath largely depends. The proper control of these muscles will result in the ability to attain the maximum degree of lung expansion, and to secure the greatest amount of the life-giving properties of the air to the system.

The Yogis classify Respiration into four general methods, *viz.*:

(1) High Breathing.

(2) Mid Breathing.

(3) Low Breathing.

(4) Yogi Complete Breathing

We will give a general idea of the first three methods, and a more extended treatment of the fourth method, upon which the Yogi Science of Breath is largely based.

(1) High Breathing

This form of breathing is known to the Western world as Clavicular Breathing, or Collarbone Breathing. One breathing in this way elevates the ribs and raises the collarbone and shoulders, at the same time drawing in the abdomen and pushing its contents up against the diaphragm, which in turn is raised.

The upper part of the chest and lungs, which is the smallest, is used, and consequently but a minimum amount of air enters the lungs. In addition to this, the diaphragm being raised, there can be no expansion in that direction. A study of the anatomy of the chest will convince any student that in this way a maximum amount of effort is used to obtain a minimum amount of benefit.

High Breathing is probably the worst form of breathing known to man and requires the greatest expenditure of energy with the smallest amount of benefit. It is an energy-wasting, poor-returns plan. It is quite common among the Western races, many women being addicted to it, and even singers, clergymen, lawyers and others, who should know better, using it ignorantly.

Many diseases of the vocal organs and organs of respiration may be directly traced to this barbarous method of breathing, and the straining of delicate organs caused by this method, often results in the harsh, disagreeable voices heard on all sides. Many persons who breathe in this way become addicted to the disgusting practice of "mouth-breathing" described in a subsequent chapter.

If the student has any doubts about what has been

said regarding this form of breathing, let him try the experiment of expelling all the air from his lungs, then standing erect, with hands at sides, let him raise the shoulders and collarbone and inhale. He will find that the amount of air inhaled is far below normal. Then let him inhale a full breath, after dropping the shoulders and collarbone, and he will receive an object lesson in breathing which he will be apt to remember much longer than he would any words, printed or spoken.

(2) Mid Breathing

This method of respiration is known to Western students as Rib Breathing, or Intercostal Breathing, and while less objectionable than High Breathing, is far inferior to either Low Breathing or to the Yogi Complete Breath. In Mid Breathing the diaphragm is pushed upward, and the abdomen drawn in. The ribs are raised somewhat, and the chest is partially expanded. It is quite common among men who have made no study of the subject. As there are two better methods known, we give it only passing notice, and that principally to call your attention to its shortcomings.

(3) Low Breathing

This form of respiration is far better than either of the two preceding forms, and of recent years many Western writers have extolled its merits, and have exploited it under the names of "Abdominal Breathing," "Deep Breathing," "Diaphragmic Breathing," etc., etc., and much good has been accomplished by the attention of the public having been directed to the subject, and many having been induced to substitute it for the inferior and injurious methods above alluded to. Many "systems" of breathing have been built around Low Breathing, and students have paid high prices to learn the new (?) systems. But, as we have said, much good has resulted and after all the students who paid high prices to learn revamped old systems undoubtedly got their money's worth if they were induced to discard the old methods of High Breathing and Low Breathing.

Although many Western authorities write and speak of this method as the best known form of breathing, the Yogis knew it to be but a part of a system which they have used for centuries and which they know as "The Complete Breath." It must be admitted, however, that one must be acquainted with the principles of Low Breathing before he can grasp the idea of Complete Breathing.

Let us again consider the diaphragm. What is it? We have seen that it is the great partition muscle, which separates the chest and its contents from the abdomen and its contents. When at rest it presents a concave surface to the abdomen. That is, the diaphragm as viewed from the abdomen would seem like the sky as viewed from the earth—the interior of an arched surface. Consequently the side of the diaphragm toward the chest organs is like a protruding rounded surface—like a hill. When the diaphragm is brought into use the hill formation is lowered and the diaphragm presses upon the abdominal organs and forces out the abdomen.

In Low Breathing, the lungs are given freer play

than in the methods already mentioned, and consequently more air is inhaled. This fact has led the majority of Western writers to speak and write of Low Breathing (which they call Abdominal Breathing) as the highest and best method known to science. But the Oriental Yogi has long known of a better method, and some few Western writers have also recognized this fact. The trouble with all methods of breathing, other than "Yogi Complete Breathing," is that in none of these methods do the lungs become filled with air—at the best only a portion of the lung space is filled, even in Low Breathing. High Breathing fills only the upper portion of the lungs. Mid Breathing fills only the middle and a portion of the upper parts. Low Breathing fills only the lower and middle parts. It is evident that any method that fills the entire lung space must be far preferable to those filling only certain parts. Any method which will fill the entire lung space must be of the greatest value to man in the way of allowing him to absorb the greatest quantity of oxygen and to store away the greatest amount of prana. The Complete Breath is known to the Yogis to be the best method of respiration known to science.

The Yogi Complete Breath

Yogi Complete Breathing includes all the good points of High Breathing, Mid Breathing and Low Breathing, with the objectionable features of each eliminated. It brings into play the entire respiratory apparatus, every part of the lungs, every air-cell, every respiratory muscle. The entire respiratory organism responds to this method of breathing, and the maximum amount of benefit is derived from the minimum expenditure of energy. The chest cavity is increased to its normal limits in all directions and every part of the machinery performs its natural work and functions.

One of the most important features of this method of breathing is the fact that the respiratory muscles are fully called into play, whereas in the other forms of breathing only a portion of these muscles are so used. In Complete Breathing, among other muscles, those controlling the ribs are actively used, which increases the space in which the lungs may expand, and also gives the proper support to the organs when needed, Nature availing herself of the perfection of the principle of leverage in this process. Certain muscles hold the lower ribs firmly in position, while other muscles bend them outward.

Then again, in this method, the diaphragm is under perfect control and is able to perform its functions properly, and in such manner as to yield the maximum degree of service.

In the rib action, above alluded to, the lower ribs are controlled by the diaphragm which draws them slightly downward, while other muscles hold them in place and the intercostal muscles force them outward, which combined action increases the mid-chest cavity to its maximum. In addition to this muscular action, the upper ribs are also lifted and forced outward by the intercostal muscles, which increases the capacity of the upper chest to its fullest extent.

If you have studied the special features of the four given methods of breathing, you will at once see that the Complete Breathing comprises all the advantageous features of the three other methods, plus the reciprocal advantages accruing from the combined action of the high-chest, mid-chest, and diaphragmic regions, and the normal rhythm thus obtained.

The Yogi Complete Breath is the fundamental breath of the entire Yogi Science of Breath, and the student must fully acquaint himself with it, and master it perfectly before he can hope to obtain results from the other forms of breath mentioned and given in this book. He should not be content with half-learning it, but should go to work in earnest until it becomes his natural method of breathing. This will require work, time and patience, but without these things nothing is ever accomplished. There is no royal road to the Science of Breath, and the student must be prepared to practise and study in earnest if he expects to receive results. The results obtained by a complete mastery of the Science of Breath are great, and no one who has attained them would willingly go back to the old methods, and he will tell his friends that he considers himself amply repaid for all his work. We say these things now, that you may fully understand the necessity and importance of mastering this fundamental method of Yogi Breathing, instead of passing it by and trying some of the attractive looking variations given later on in this book. Again, we say to you: Start right, and right results will follow; but neglect your foundations and your entire building will topple over sooner or later.

Perhaps the better way to teach you how to develop the Yogi Complete Breath would be to give you simple directions regarding the breath itself, and then follow up the same with general remarks concerning it, and then later on giving exercises for developing the chest, muscles and lungs which have been allowed to remain in an undeveloped condition by imperfect methods of breathing. Right here we wish to say that this Complete Breath is not a forced or abnormal thing, but on the contrary is a going back to first principles—a return to Nature. The healthy adult savage and the healthy infant of civilization both breathe in this manner, but civilized man has adopted unnatural methods of living, clothing, etc., and has lost his birthright. And we wish to remind the reader that the Complete Breath does not necessarily call for the complete filling of the lungs at every inhalation. One may inhale the average amount of air, using the Complete Breathing Method and distributing the air inhaled, be the quantity large or small, to all parts of the lungs. But one should inhale a series of full Complete Breaths several times a day, whenever opportunity offers, in order to keep the system in good order and condition.

The following simple exercise will give you a clear idea of what the Complete Breath is :

(1) Stand or sit erect. Breathing through the nostrils, inhale steadily, first filling the lower part of the lungs, which is accomplished by bringing into play the diaphragm, which descending exerts a gentle pressure on the abdominal organs, pushing forward the front walls of the abdomen. Then fill the middle part of the lungs, pushing out the lower ribs, breastbone and chest. Then fill the higher

portion of the lungs, protruding the upper chest, thus lifting the chest, including the upper six or seven pairs of ribs. In the final movement, the lower part of the abdomen will be slightly drawn in, which movement gives the lungs a support and also helps to fill the highest part of the lungs.

At first reading it may appear that this breath consists of three distinct movements. This, however, is not the correct idea. The inhalation is continuous, the entire chest cavity from the lowered diaphragm to the highest point of the chest in the region of the collarbone, being expanded with a uniform movement. Avoid a jerky series of inhalations, and strive to attain a steady continuous action. Practice will soon overcome the tendency to divide the inhalation into three movements, and will result in a uniform continuous breath. You will be able to complete the inhalation in a couple of seconds after a little practice.

(2) Retain the breath a few seconds.

(3) Exhale quite slowly, holding the chest in a firm position, and drawing the abdomen in a little and lifting it upward slowly as the air leaves the lungs. When the air is entirely exhaled, relax the chest and abdomen. A little practice will render this part of the exercise easy, and the movement once acquired will be afterwards performed almost automatically.

It will be seen that by this method of breathing all parts of the respiratory apparatus is brought into action, and all parts of the lungs, including the most remote air cells, are exercised. The chest cavity is expanded in all directions. You will also notice that the Complete Breath is really a combination of Low, Mid and High Breaths, succeeding each other rapidly in the order given, in such a manner as to form one uniform, continuous, complete breath.

You will find it quite a help to you if you will practise this breath before a large mirror, placing the hands lightly over the abdomen so that you may feel the movements. At the end of the inhalation, it is well to occasionally slightly elevate the shoulders, thus raising the collarbone and allowing the air to pass freely into the small upper lobe of the right lung, which place is sometimes the breeding place of tuberculosis.

At the beginning of practice, you may have more or less trouble in acquiring the Complete Breath, but a little practice will make perfect, and when you have once acquired it you will never willingly return to the old methods.

CHAPTER XV

EFFECT OF CORRECT BREATHING

SCARCELY too much can be said of the advantages attending the practice of the Complete Breath. And yet the student who has carefully read the foregoing pages should scarcely need to have pointed out to him such advantages.

The practice of the Complete Breath will make any man or woman immune to Consumption and other pulmonary troubles, and will do away with all liability to contract "colds," as well as bronchial and similar weaknesses. Consumption is due principally to lowered vitality attributable to an insufficient amount of air being inhaled. The impairment of vitality renders the system open to attacks from disease germs. Imperfect breathing allows a considerable part of the lungs to remain inactive, and such portions offer an inviting field for bacilli, which invading the weakened tissue soon produce havoc. Good, healthy lung tissue will resist the germs, and the only way to have good, healthy lung tissue is to use the lungs properly.

Consumptives are nearly all narrow-chested. What does this mean? Simply that these people were addicted to improper habits of breathing, and consequently their chests failed to develop and expand. The man who practises the Complete Breath will have a full, broad chest, and the narrow-chested man may develop his chest to normal proportions if he will but adopt this mode of breathing. Such people must develop their chest cavities if they value their lives. Colds may often be prevented by practising a little vigorous Complete Breathing whenever you feel that you are being unduly exposed. When chilled, breathe vigorously a few minutes, and you will feel a glow all over your body. Most colds can be cured by Complete Breathing and partial fasting for a day.

The quality of the blood depends largely upon its proper oxygenation in the lungs, and if it is under-oxygenated it becomes poor in quality and laden with all sorts of impurities, and the system suffers from lack of nourishment and often becomes actually poisoned by the waste products remaining unelim-inated in the blood. As the entire body, every organ and every part, is dependent upon the blood for nourishment, impure blood must have a serious effect upon the entire system. The remedy is plain—practise the Yogi Complete Breath.

The stomach and other organs of nutrition suffer much from improper breathing. Not only are they ill nourished by reason of the lack of oxygen, but as the food must absorb oxygen from the blood and become oxygenated before it can be digested and assimilated, it is readily seen how digestion and assimilation are impaired by incorrect breathing. And whenever assimilation is not normal, the system receives less and less nourishment, the appetite fails, bodily vigour decreases, and energy diminishes, and the man withers and declines. All from the lack of proper breathing.

Even the nervous system suffers from improper

breathing, inasmuch as the brain, the spinal cord, the nerve centres, and the nerves themselves, when improperly nourished by means of the blood, become poor and inefficient instruments for generating, storing and transmitting the nerve currents. And improperly nourished they will become if sufficient oxygen is not absorbed through the lungs. There is another aspect of the case whereby the nerve currents themselves, or rather the force from which the nerve currents spring, becomes lessened from want of proper breathing, but this belongs to another phase of the subject which is treated of in other chapters of this book, and our purpose here is tc direct your attention to the fact that the mechanism of the nervous system is rendered inefficient as an instrument for conveying nerve force, as the indirect result of a lack of proper breathing.

In the practice of the Complete Breath, during inhalation, the diaphragm contracts and exerts a gentle pressure upon the liver, stomach and other organs, which in connection with the rhythm of the lungs acts as a gentle massage of these organs and stimulates their actions, and encourages normal functioning. Each inhalation aids in this internal exercise, and assists in causing a normal circulation to the organs of nutrition and elimination. In High or Mid Breathing the organs lose the benefit accruing from this internal massage.

The Western world is paying much attention to Physical Culture just now, which is a good thing. But in their enthusiasm they must not forget that the exercise of the external muscles is not everything. The internal organs also need exercise, and Nature's plan for this exercise is proper breathing. The diaphragm is Nature's principal instrument for this internal exercise. Its motion vibrates the important organs of nutrition and elimination, and massages and kneads them at each inhalation and exhalation, forcing blood into them, and then squeezing it out, and imparting a general tone to the organs. Any organ or part of the body which is not exercised gradually atrophies and refuses to function properly, and lack of the internal exercise afforded by the diaphragmatic action leads to diseased organs. The Complete Breath gives the proper motion to the diaphragm, as well as exercising the middle and upper chest. It is indeed " complete " in its action.

From the standpoint of Western physiology alone, without reference to the Oriental philosophies and science, this Yogi system of Complete Breathing is of vital importance to every man, woman and child who wishes to acquire health and keep it. Its very simplicity keeps thousands from seriously considering it, while they spend fortunes in seeking health through complicated and expensive "systems." Health knocks at their door and they answer not. Verily the stone which the builders reject is the real cornerstone of the Temple of Health.

CHAPTER XVI

BREATHING EXERCISES

WE give below three forms of breath, quite popular among the Yogis. The first is the well-known Yogi Cleansing Breath, to which is attributed much of the great lung endurance found among the Yogis. They usually finish up a breathing exercise with this Cleansing Breath, and we have followed this plan in this book. We also give the Yogi Nerve Vitalizing Exercise, which has been handed down among them for ages, and which has never been improved on by Western teachers of Physical Culture, although some of them have " borrowed " it from teachers of Yogi. We also give the Yogi Vocal Breath, which accounts largely for the melodious, vibrant voices of the better class of the Oriental Yogis. We feel that if this book contained nothing more than these three exercises, it would be invaluable to the Western student. Take these exercises as a gift from your Eastern brothers and put them into practice.

THE YOGI CLEANSING BREATH

The Yogis have a favourite form of breathing which they practise when they feel the necessity of ventilating and cleansing the lungs. They conclude many of their other breathing exercises with this breath, and we have followed this practice in this book. This Cleansing Breathing ventilates and cleanses the lungs, stimulates the cells and gives a general tone to the respiratory organs, and is conducive to their general healthy condition. Besides this effect, it is found to greatly refresh the entire system. Speakers, singers, etc., will find this breath especially restful, after having tired the respiratory organs.

(1) Inhale a complete breath.

(2) Retain the air a few seconds.

(3) Pucker up the lips as if for a whistle (but do not swell out the cheeks), then exhale a little air through the opening, with considerable vigour. Then stop for a moment, retaining the air, and then exhale a little more air. Repeat until the air is completely exhaled. Remember that considerable vigour is to be used in exhaling the air through the opening in the lips.

This breath will be found quite refreshing when one is tired and generally "used up." A trial will convince the student of its merits. This exercise should be practised until it can be performed naturally, and easily, as it is used to finish up a number of other exercises given in this book, and it should be thoroughly understood.

The Yogi Nerve Vitalizing Breath

This is an exercise well known to the Yogis, who consider it one of the strongest nerve stimulants and invigorants known to man. Its purpose is to stimulate the Nervous System, develop nerve force, energy and vitality. This exercise brings a stimulating pressure to bear on important nerve centres, which in turn stimulate and energize the entire nervous system, and send an increased flow of nerve force to all parts of the body.

(1) Stand erect.

(2) Inhale a Complete Breath, and retain same.

(3) Extend the arms straight in front of you, letting them be somewhat limp and relaxed, with only sufficient nerve force to hold them out.

(4) Slowly draw the hands back toward the shoulders, gradually contracting the muscles and putting force into them, so that when they reach the shoulders the fists will be so tightly clenched that a tremulous motion is felt.

(5) Then, keeping the muscles tense, push the fists slowly out, and then draw them back rapidly (still tense) several times.

(6) Exhale vigorously through the mouth.

(7) Practise the Cleansing Breath.

The efficiency of this exercise depends greatly upon the speed of the drawing back of the fists, and the tension of the muscles, and, of course, upon the full lungs. This exercise must be tried to be appreciated. It is without equal as a "bracer," as our Western friends put it.

The Yogi Vocal Breath

The Yogis have a form of breathing to develop the voice. They are noted for their wonderful voices, which are strong, smooth and clear, and have a wonderful trumpet-like carrying power. They have practised this particular form of breathing exercise which has resulted in rendering their voices soft, beautiful and flexible, imparting to it that indescribable, peculiar floating quality, combined with great power. The exercise given below will in time impart the above-mentioned qualities, or the Yogi Voice, to the student who practises it faithfully. It is to be understood, of course, that this form of breath is to be used only as an occasional exercise, and not as a regular form of breathing.

(1) Inhale a Complete Breath very slowly, but steadily, through the nostrils, taking as much time as possible in the inhalation.

(2) Retain for a few seconds.

(3) Expel the air vigorously in one great breath, through the wide opened mouth.

(4) Rest the lungs by the Cleansing Breath.

Without going deeply into the Yogi theories of sound-production in speaking and singing, we wish to say that experience has taught them that the timbre, quality and power of a voice depend not alone upon the vocal organs in the throat, but that the facial muscles, etc., have much to do with the matter. Some men with large chests produce but a poor tone, while others with comparatively small chests produce tones of amazing strength and quality. Here is an interesting experiment worth trying: Stand before a glass and pucker up your mouth and whistle, and note the shape of your mouth and the general expression of your face. Then sing or speak as you do naturally, and see the difference. Then start to whistle again for a few seconds, and then, *without changing the position of your lips or face*, sing a few notes and notice what a vibrant, resonant, clear and beautiful tone is produced.

The following are the seven favourite exercises of the Yogis for developing the lungs, muscles, ligaments, air cells, etc. They are quite simple but marvellously effective. Do not let the simplicity of these exercises make you lose interest, for they are the result of careful experiments and practice on the part of the Yogis, and are the essence of numerous intricate and complicated exercises, the non-essential portions being eliminated and the essential features retained.

(1) The Retained Breath

This is a very important exercise which tends to strengthen and develop the respiratory muscles as well as the lungs, and its frequent practice will also tend to expand the chest. The Yogis have found that an occasional holding of the breath, after the lungs have been filled with the Complete Breath, is very beneficial, not only to the respiratory organs but to the organs of nutrition, the nervous system, and the blood itself. They have found that an occasional holding of the breath tends to purify the air which has remained in the lungs from former inhalations, and to more fully oxygenate the blood. They also know that the breath so retained gathers up all the waste matter, and when the breath is expelled it carries with it the effete matter of the system, and cleanses the lungs just as a purgative does the bowels. The Yogis recommend this exercise for various disorders of the stomach, liver and blood, and also find that it frequently relieves bad breath, which often arises from poorly ventilated lungs. We recommend students to pay considerable attention to this exercise, as it has great merits. The following directions will give you a clear idea of the exercise:

(1) Stand erect.

(2) Inhale a Complete Breath.

(3) Retain the air as long as you can comfortably.

(4) Exhale vigorously through the open mouth.

(5) Practise the Cleansing Breath.

At first you will be able to retain the breath only a short time, but a little practice will also show a great improvement. Time yourself with a watch if you wish to note your progress.

(2) Lung Cell Stimulation

This exercise is designed to stimulate the air cells in the lungs, but beginners must not overdo it, and in no case should it be indulged in too vigorously. Some may find a slight dizziness resulting from the first few trials, in which case let them walk around a little and discontinue the exercise for a while.

(1) Stand erect, with hands at sides.

(2) Breathe in very slowly, and gradually.

(3) While inhaling, gently tap the chest with the finger tips, constantly changing position.

(4) When the lungs are filled, retain the breath and pat the chest with the palms of the hands.

(5) Practise the Cleansing Breath.

This exercise is very bracing and stimulating to the whole body, and is a well-known Yogi practice. Many of the air cells of the lungs become inactive by reason of incomplete breathing, and often become almost atrophied. One who has practised imperfect breathing for years will find it not so easy to stimulate all these ill-used air cells into activity all at once by the Complete Breath, but this exercise will do much toward bringing about the desired result, and is worth study and practice.

(3) Rib Stretching

We have explained that the ribs are fastened by cartilages, which admit of considerable expansion. In proper breathing, the ribs play an important part, and it is well to occasionally give them a little special exercise in order to preserve their elasticity. Standing or sitting in unnatural positions, to which many of the Western people are addicted, is apt to render the ribs more or less stiff and inelastic, and this exercise will do much to overcome same.

(1) Stand erect.

(2) Place the hands one on each side of the body, as high up under the armpits as convenient, the thumbs reaching toward the back, the palms on the side of the chest and fingers to the front over the breast.

(3) Inhale a Complete Breath.

(4) Retain the air for a short time.

(5) Then gently squeeze the sides, at the same time slowly exhaling.

(6) Practise the Cleansing Breath.

Use moderation in this exercise and do not overdo it.

(4) Chest Expansion

The chest is quite apt to be contracted from bending over one's work. This exercise is very good for the purpose of restoring natural conditions and gaining chest expansion.

(1) Stand erect.

(2) Inhale a Complete Breath.

(3) Retain the air.

(4) Extend both arms forward and bring the two clenched fists together on a level with the shoulder.

(5) Then swing back the fists vigorously until the arms stand out straight sideways from the shoulders.

(6) Then bring back to Position 4, and swing to Position 5. Repeat several times.

(7) Exhale vigorously through the opened mouth.

(8) Practise the Cleansing Breath.

Use moderation and do not overdo this exercise.

(5) Walking Exercise

(1) Walk with head up, chin drawn slightly in, shoulders back, and with measured tread.

(2) Inhale a Complete Breath, counting (mentally) 1, 2, 3, 4, 5, 6, 7, 8, one count to each step, making the inhalation extend over the eight counts.

(3) Exhale slowly, through the nostrils, counting as before—1, 2, 3, 4, 5, 6, 7, 8—one count to a step.

(4) Rest between breaths, continuing walking and counting, 1, 2, 3, 4, 5, 6, 7, 8, one count to the step.

(5) Repeat until you begin to feel tired. Then rest for a while, and resume at pleasure. Repeat several times a day.

Some Yogis vary this exercise by retaining the breath during a 1, 2, 3, 4, count, and then exhale in an eight-step count. Practise whichever plan seems most agreeable to you.

(6) Morning Exercise

(1) Stand erect in a military attitude, head up, eyes front, shoulders back, knees stiff, hands at sides.

(2) Raise body slowly on toes, inhaling a Complete Breath, steadily and slowly.

(3) Retain the breath for a few seconds, maintaining the same position.

(4) Slowly sink to the first position, at the same time slowly exhaling the air through the nostrils.

(5) Practise Cleansing Breath.

(6) Repeat several times, varying by using right leg alone, then left leg alone.

(7) Stimulating Circulation

(1) Stand erect.

(2) Inhale a Complete Breath and retain.

(3) Bend forward slightly and grasp a stick or cane steadily and firmly, and gradually exerting your entire strength upon the grasp.

(4) Relax the grasp, return to first position, and slowly exhale.

(5) Repeat several times.

(6) Finish with the Cleansing Breath.

This exercise may be performed without the use of a stick or cane, by grasping an imaginary cane, using the will to exert the pressure. The exercise is a favourite Yogi plan of stimulating the circulation by driving the arterial blood to the extremities, and drawing back the venous blood to the heart and lungs that it may take up the oxygen which has been inhaled with the air. In cases of poor circulation there is not enough blood in the lungs to absorb the increased amount of oxygen inhaled, and the system does not get the full benefit of the improved breathing. In such cases, particularly, it is well to practise this exercise, occasionally with the regular Complete Breathing Exercise.

CHAPTER XVII

NOSTRIL-BREATHING VS. MOUTH-BREATHING

One of the first lessons in the Yogi Science of Breath is to learn how to breathe through the nostrils, and to overcome the common practice of mouth-breathing.

The breathing mechanism of man is so constructed that he may breathe either through the mouth or nasal tubes, but it is a matter of vital importance to him which method he follows, as one brings health and strength and the other disease and weakness.

It should not be necessary to state to the student that the proper method of breathing is to take the breath through the nostrils, but alas! the ignorance among civilized people regarding this simple matter is astounding. We find people in all walks of life habitually breathing through their mouths, and allowing their children to follow their horrible and disgusting example.

Many of the diseases to which civilized man is subject are undoubtedly caused by this common habit of mouth-breathing. Children permitted to breathe in this way grow up with impaired vitality and weakened constitutions, and in manhood and womanhood break down and become chronic invalids. The mother of the savage race does better, being evidently guided by her intuition. She seems to instinctively recognize that the nostrils are the proper channels for the conveyal of air to the lungs, and she trains her infant to close its little lips and breathe through the nose. She tips its head forward when it is asleep, which attitude closes the lips and makes nostril breathing imperative. If our civilized mothers were to adopt the same plan, it would work a great good for the race.

Many contagious diseases are contracted by the disgusting habit of mouth-breathing, and many cases of cold and catarrhal affections are also attributable to the same cause. Many persons who, for the sake of appearances, keep their mouth closed during the day, persist in mouth-breathing at night and often contract disease in this way. Carefully conducted scientific experiments have shown that soldiers and sailors who sleep with their mouths open are much more liable to contract contagious diseases than those who breathe properly through the nostrils. An instance is related in which small-pox became epidemic on a man-of-war in foreign parts, and every death which resulted was that of some sailor or marine who was a mouth-breather, not a single nostril-breather succumbing.

The organs of respiration have their only protective apparatus, filter, or dust-catcher, in the nostrils. When the breath is taken through the mouth, there is nothing from mouth to lungs to strain the air, or to catch the dust and other foreign matter in the air. From mouth to lungs the dirt or impure substance has a clear track, and the entire respiratory system is unprotected. And, moreover, such incorrect breathing admits cold air to the organs, thereby injuring them. Inflammation of the respiratory organs often results from the inhalation of cold air through the mouth. The man who breathes through the mouth at night, always awakens with a parched feeling in the mouth and a dryness in the throat. He is violating one of nature's laws, and is sowing the seeds of disease.

Once more, remember that the mouth affords no protection to the respiratory organs, and cold air, dust and impurities and germs readily enter by that door. On the other hand, the nostrils and nasal passages show evidence of the careful design of nature in this respect. The nostrils are two narrow, tortuous channels, containing numerous bristly hairs which serve the purpose of a filter or sieve to strain the air of its impurities, etc., which are expelled when the breath is exhaled. Not only do the nostrils serve this important purpose, but they also perform an important function in warming the air inhaled. The long narrow winding nostrils are filled with warm mucous membrane, which coming in contact with the inhaled air warms it, so that it can do no damage to the delicate organs of the throat, or to the lungs.

No animal, excepting man, sleeps with the mouth open or breathes through the mouth, and in fact it is believed that it is only civilized man who so perverts nature's functions, as the savage and barbarian races almost invariably breathe correctly. It is probable that this unnatural habit among civilized men has been acquired through unnatural methods of living, enervating luxuries and excessive warmth.

The refining, filtering and straining apparatus of the nostrils renders the air fit to reach the delicate organs of the throat and the lungs, and the air is not fit to so reach these organs until it has passed through nature's refining process. The impurities which are stopped and retained by the sieves and mucous membrane of the nostrils, are thrown out again by the expelled breath, in exhalation, and in case they have accumulated too rapidly, or have managed to escape through the sieves and have penetrated forbidden regions, nature protects us by producing a sneeze which violently ejects the intruder.

The air, when it enters the lungs, is as different from the outside air, as is distilled water different from the water of the cistern. The intricate purifying organization of the nostrils, arresting and holding the impure particles in the air, is as important as is the action of the mouth in stopping cherry stones and fish bones and preventing them from being carried on to the stomach. Man should no more breathe through his mouth than he would attempt to take food through his nose.

Another feature of mouth-breathing is that the nasal passages, being thus comparatively unused, consequently fail to keep themselves clean and clear, and become clogged up and unclean, and are apt to contract local diseases. Like abandoned roads that soon become filled with weeds and rubbish, unused nostrils become filled with impurities and foul matter.

One who habitually breathes through the nostrils is not likely to be troubled with clogged or stuffy nostrils, but for the benefit of those who have been more or less addicted to the unnatural mouth-breathing, and who wish to acquire the natural and rational method, it may perhaps be well to add a few words regarding the way to keep their nostrils clean and free from impurities.

A favourite Oriental method is to snuff a little water up the nostrils allowing it to run down the passage into the throat, from thence it may be ejected through the mouth. Some Hindu Yogis immerse the face in a bowl of water, but this latter method requires considerable practice, and the first mentioned method is equally efficacious, and much more easily performed.

Another good plan is to open the window and breathe freely, closing one nostril with the finger or thumb, sniffing up the air through the open nostril. Then repeat the process on the other nostril. Repeat several times, changing nostrils. This method will usually clear the nostrils of obstructions.

We urge upon the student the necessity of acquiring this method of breathing if he has it not, and caution him against dismissing this phase of the subject as unimportant.

CHAPTER XVIII

THE LITTLE LIVES OF THE BODY

HATHA YOGA teaches that the physical body is built up of cells, each cell containing within it a miniature "life" which controls its action. These "lives" are really bits of intelligent mind of a certain degree of development, which enable the cells to do their work properly. These bits of intelligence are, of course, subordinate to the control of the central mind of man, and readily obey orders given from headquarters, consciously or unconsciously. These cell intelligences manifest a perfect adaption for their particular work. The selective action of the cells, extracting from the blood the nourishment required, and rejecting that which is not needed is an instance of this intelligence. The process of digestion, assimilation, etc., shows the intelligence of the cells, either separately or collectively, in groups. The healing of wounds, the rush of the cells to the points where they are most needed, and hundreds of other examples known to the investigators, all mean to the Yogi student examples of the "life" within each atom. Each atom is to the Yogi a living thing, leading its own independent life. These atoms combine into groups for some end, and the groups manifest a group-intelligence, so long as it remains a group; these groups again combining in turn, and forming bodies of a more complex nature, which serve as vehicles for higher forms of consciousness.

When death comes to the physical body, the cells separate and scatter and that which we call decay sets in. The force which has held the cells together is withdrawn, and they become free to go their own way and to form new combinations. Some go into the body of the plants in the vicinity, and eventually find themselves in the body of an animal; others remain in the organism of the plant; others remain in the ground for a time, but the life of the atom means incessant and constant change. As a leading writer has said: "Death is but an aspect of life, and the destruction of one material form is but a prelude to the building up of another." We will give our students a brief idea of the nature and work of this cell-life—the life of these little lives of the body.

The cells of the body have three principles: (1) Matter, which they obtain from the food; (2) Prana, or vital force, which enables them to manifest action, and which is obtained from the food we eat; the water we drink and the air we breathe; (3) Intelligence, or "mind-stuff," which is obtained from the Universal Mind. We will first take up the material side of cell-life.

As we have said, every living body is a collection of minute cells. This is, of course, true of every part of the body, from the hard bone to the softest tissue—from the enamel of the tooth to the most delicate part of the mucous membrane. These cells have different shapes, which are regulated by the requirements of its particular office, or work. Each cell is, to all intents and purposes, an individual, separate and more or less independent, although subject to the control of cell-group mind ; large group commands ; and, finally, to the central mind of the man, the controlling work, or at least the greater part of it, coming within the control of the Instinctive Mind.

These cells are constantly at work, performing all the duties of the body, each having its own particular work to do—and doing it to the best of its ability. Some of the cells belong to the " reserves " and are kept under " waiting orders " ready for some sudden demand of duty. Others belong to the army of active workers of the cell-community and manufacture the secretions and fluids needed in the varied work of the system. Some of the cells are stationary —others remain so until needed, when they manifest motion—others are constantly on the move, some making regular trips and some being rovers. Of these moving cells some perform the work of carriers, some move from place to place doing odd jobs, and others do scavenger work, and still another class belong to the police force, or army, of the cell-community. Cell-life in the body may be compared to a large colony, operated on a co-operative plan, each cell having its own work to do for the common good, each working for all, and all working for the common welfare. The cells of the nervous system carry messages from one part of the body to the brain and from the brain to another part of the body, being living telegraph wires, as the nerves are composed of minute cells in close contact with each other, having small projections which are in contact with similar projections from other cells, so that they are practically holding hands and forming a chain, along which passes the Prana.

Of the carriers, moving workers, policemen, soldiers, etc., of the cell-community there are millions upon millions in each human body, it being estimated that there are in one cubic inch of blood at least 75,000,000,000 (seventy-five thousand million) of the red-blood cells alone, not to speak of the other cells. The community is a large one.

The red-blood cells, which are the common carriers of the body, float in the arteries and veins, taking up a load of oxygen from the lungs and carrying it to the various tissues of the body, giving life and strength to the parts. On the return journey through the veins they carry with them the waste products of the system, which are then thrown off by the lungs, etc. Like a merchant vessel these cells carry a cargo on their out-going trip and bring a second cargo on their return trip. Other cells force their way through the walls of the arteries and veins and through the tissues on their errand of repair work, etc., upon which they have been sent.

Besides the red-blood cells, or carriers, there are several other kinds of cells in the blood. Among the most interesting of these are the policemen and soldiers of the cell-community. The work of these cells is to protect the system from germs, bacteria, etc., which might cause trouble or disease. When one of these policemen comes in contact with an intruding germ, the police cell enmeshes it and then proceeds to devour it, if it be not too large—if it be too large for him to get away with he summons other cells to his assistance, when the combined force gather around the enemy and carry it to some point of the body where it may be thrown out. Boils, pimples, etc., are instances of the throwing out of some intruding enemy or enemies by these policemen of the system.

There is much work for the red-blood cells to do. They carry the oxygen to the parts of the body; they push along the nourishment obtained from the food to the parts of the body where it is needed to build up and repair; they extract from the nourishment just the elements needed to manufacture gastric juice, saliva, pancreatic juices, bile, milk, etc., etc., and then combine them in the proper proportions for use. They do a thousand and one things and are busy continuously like a lot of ants in and around an anthill. The Oriental teachers have long known and taught of the existence and work of these "little lives," but it has remained for Western science to dig into the subject in such a way as to bring to light the details of their work.

Cells are being born and cells are dying every moment of our existence. Cells reproduce themselves by enlarging and subdividing, the original cell swelling until it finally forms two parts with a small connecting "waist"; then the connection parts and there are two independent cells instead of one. The new cell in turn divides itself up, and so on.

Cells enable the body to carry on its work of continual regeneration. Every part of the human body is undergoing a constant change and tissues are being continually renewed. Our skin, bones, hair, muscles, etc., are constantly being repaired and "made over." It takes about four months to replace our finger nails—about four weeks to replace our skin. Every part of our bodies is being worn out and renewed and repaired constantly. And these little workmen—the cells—are the agency performing this wonderful task. Millions of these little workers are ever moving along or working in a fixed position in all parts of our bodies, renewing the worn-out tissues and replacing them with new material and throwing out of the system the worn-out and injurious particles of matter.

In the lower animals Nature allows the Instinctive Mind a fuller scope and a larger field, and as life ascends in the scale, developing the reasoning faculties, the Instinctive Mind seems to narrow its field. For instance, crabs and members of the spider family are able to grow new feeders, legs, claws, etc. Snails are able to grow even parts of the head, including eyes, which have been destroyed; some fishes are able to regrow tails. Salamanders and lizards are able to grow new tails, including bones, muscle and parts of the spinal column. The very lowest forms of animal life have practically an unlimited power of restoring lost parts and can practically make themselves entirely over, provided there is left the smallest part of them to build upon. The higher form of animals have lost much of this recuperative power and man has lost more than any of them owing to his mode of living. Some of the more advanced of the Hatha Yogis, however, have performed some wonderful results along these lines, and anyone, with patient practice, may obtain such control of the Instinctive Mind and the cells under its control that he may obtain wonderful recuperative results in the direction of renewing diseased parts and weakened portions of the body.

But even ordinary man still possesses a wonderful degree of recuperative power, which is constantly being manifested, although the average man pays no attention to it. Let us take the healing of a wound for example. Let us see how it is performed. It is well worth your consideration and study. It is so common that we are apt to overlook it, and yet so wonderful as to cause the student to realize the greatness of the intelligence displayed and called into force in the work.

Let us suppose that a human body is wounded—that is, cut or torn by some outside agency. The tissues, lymphatic and blood-vessels, glands, muscles, nerves, and sometimes even the bone, are severed, and the continuity interrupted. The wound bleeds, gapes and causes pain. The nerves carry the message to the brain, calling loudly for immediate help, and the Instinctive Mind sends messages here and there in the body, calling out a sufficient force of repair workmen, who are hurried to the scene of danger. In the meantime the blood pouring from the injured blood-vessels washes away, or at least tries to wash away, the foreign substances that have entered the organism, such as dirt, bacteria, etc., which would act as poisons if allowed to remain. The blood, coming in contact with the outside air, coagulates and forms a sticky sort of substance, somewhat resembling glue, and forms the beginning of the coming crust or scab. The millions of blood cells whose duty it is to do the repair work arrive on the scene on the " double-quick " and at once begin to again connect the tissues, displaying the most wonderful intelligence and activity in their work. The cells of the tissues, nerves, blood-vessels, on both sides of the wound, begin to increase and multiply, bringing into being millions of new cells, which, advancing from both sides, finally meet in the centre of the wound. This forming of new cells bears all the appearance of a disorderly, purposeless effort, but in a short time the hand of the commanding intelligence and of its subordinate centres of influence begins to show itself. The new cells of the blood-vessels connect with the same kind of cells on the opposite side of the wound, forming new tubes through which the blood may flow. The cells of what is known as the "connective tissue" unite with others of their kind and draw together the wound. New nerve cells form on each of the severed ends, and, sending out filaments, gradually repair the broken wires, until at last the message passes again without interruption. After all this "inside" work is completed and blood-vessel, nerve and connective tissue are fully repaired, the cells of the skin start in to finish the task, and new epidermis cells spring into existence and new skin is formed over the wound, which has healed by that time. All orderly, showing discipline and intelligence. The healing of a wound—apparently so simple—brings the careful observer face to face with the Intelligence which pervades all of Nature—lets him see Creation in active operation. Nature is ever willing to draw aside the veil and allow us to peep a little into the sacred chamber beyond; but we poor ignorant creatures heed not her invitation, but pass by unheeding and waste our mind force on silly things and hurtful pursuits.

So much for the work of the cell. The cell-mind is supplied from the Universal Mind—the great storehouse of " mind-stuff "—and is kept in touch and directed by the mind of the cell-centres, which are in turn controlled by higher centres, until the central Instinctive Mind is reached. But the cell-mind is not able to express itself without both of two other principles—matter and prana. It needs the fresh material supplied by the well-digested food, in order to make for itself a medium of expression. It also needs a supply of prana, or vital force, in order to move and have action. The triune principle of Life —mind, matter and force—is necessary in the cell as in the man. Mind needs force or energy (prana) in order to manifest itself in action through matter. As in great things, so in small—as above, so below.

In our previous chapters we have spoken of the digestion and of the importance of giving the blood a goodly supply of nourishing, well-digested food, in order that it might properly perform its work of repairing and building up the parts of the body. In this chapter we have shown you how the cells use the material in order to do the building—how they use the material to build up themselves, and then how they *build themselves* in the body. Remember, the cells, which are used as building bricks, surround themselves with the material obtained from the food, making themselves bodies, as it were ; then take up a supply of prana or vital energy and are then carried or pushed to where they are needed, where they build themselves, and are built up into new tissue, bone, muscle, etc. Without proper material with which to form themselves bodies these cells cannot carry out their mission; in fact, cannot exist. Persons who have allowed themselves to "run down" and who are suffering from imperfect nutrition have not nearly the normal amount of blood-cells and are consequently unable to have the work of the system properly carried on. The cells must have material with which to make bodies, and there is only one way in which they can receive this material—by means of nourishment in the food. And unless there is sufficient prana in the system these cells cannot manifest sufficient energy to do their work and lack of vitality is manifested throughout the whole system.

Sometimes the Instinctive Mind is so badgered and brow-beaten by the Intellect of Man that it takes on the absurd notions and fears of the latter and fails to perform its accustomed work properly, and the cells are not properly generalled. In such cases, when the Intellect once grasps the true idea, it seeks to repair its past mistakes and begins to reassure the Instinctive Mind that it understands its duties thoroughly and will be allowed to govern its own kingdom hereafter, and this is followed up with words of encouragement and praise and confidence until the Instinctive Mind recovers its equilibrium and again manages its own household. Sometimes the Instinctive Mind has been so influenced by the previous adverse notions of its owner, or by those of outsiders, that it is so confused that it takes a long time to recover its normal poise and control. And in such cases it often seems that some of the subordinate cell-centres have practically rebelled and refuse to again submit to dictation from headquarters. In both of these cases the determined commands of the will are needed to bring about peace and order and proper work in all parts of the body. Remember that there is some form of Intelligence in every organ and part and a good strong command from the Will will generally bring about an improvement in abnormal conditions.

CHAPTER XIX

THE CONTROL OF THE INVOLUNTARY SYSTEM

In the preceding chapter of this book we have explained to you that the human body is made of millions of tiny cells, each endowed with sufficient matter to enable it to do its work—with sufficient Prana to give it the energy it requires—with sufficient "mind-stuff" to give it the degree of intelligence with which to direct its work. Each cell belongs to a cell-group or family, and the intelligence of the cell is in close rapport with the intelligence of every other cell in the group or family, the combined intelligence of the cell-group resulting in a group-mind. These groups in turn are each a part of some other larger group of groups, and so on until the whole forms a great republic of cell-mind under the direction and control of the Instinctive Mind. The control of these great groups is one of the duties of the Instinctive Mind, and it usually does its work well, unless interfered with by the Intellect, which sometimes sends it fear-thoughts and in this and other ways demoralizes the Instinctive Mind. Its work is also sometimes retarded by the Intellect insisting that it take up foreign and strange habits of regulating the physical body through the cell intelligence. For instance, in the case of constipation, the Intellect being busy with other work, will not allow the body to respond to the calls of the Instinctive Mind, acting in response to a demand from the cells of the Colon—nor does it pay attention to the demands for water—and the consequence is that the Instinctive Mind is unable to execute the proper orders, and both it and certain of the cell-groups become demoralized and scarcely know what to do—bad habits springing up and replacing the natural habit. Sometimes something akin to a rebellion springs up in some of the cell-groups, resulting no doubt from some interruption in the natural course of their government, the introduction of strange customs causing a confusion. At times it seems that some of the smaller groups (and even some of the larger on certain occasions) go on "a strike," rebelling against unaccustomed and improper work forced upon them—working overtime—and similar causes, such as a lack of proper nourishment. These little cells often act just as would men under the same circumstances—the analogy is often startling to the observer and investigator. These rebellions, or strikes, seem to spread if matters are not arranged, and even when matters are patched up the cells seem to return to their work in a sullen manner, and instead of doing the best they know how they will do as little as possible, and just when they feel like it. A restoration of normal conditions, resulting from increased nutrition, proper attention, etc., will gradually bring about a return to normal conditions, but matters may be expedited by giving the cell-groups direct orders from the Will. It is astonishing how soon order and discipline may be restored in this manner. The higher Yogis have a wonderful control over the involuntary system and can act directly upon nearly every cell in their body. And even some of the so-called Yogis of the cities of India—those little more than mountebanks, who exhibit their performances for so many coppers from each wandering traveller—are able to give interesting exhibitions of this control, some of the exhibitions, however, being disgusting to persons of fine sensibilities and painful to the real Yogis, who mourn to see a noble science prostituted in this way.

The trained will is able to act directly upon these cells and groups by a simple process of direct concentration, but this plan requires much training on the part of the student. There are other plans whereby the will is called into operation by the student repeating certain words in order to focus his Will. The auto-suggestions and affirmations of the Western world act in this way. The words focus the attention and Will upon the centre of the trouble and gradually order is restored among the striking cells, a supply of Prana also being projected to the seat of the trouble, thus giving the cells additional energy. At the same time the circulation to the affected region is increased, thereby giving the cells more nourishment and building material.

One of the simplest plans of reaching the seat of trouble and giving a vigorous order to the cells is the one taught by the Hatha Yogis to their students, to be used by them until they are able to use the concentrated Will without any aids. The plan is simply to " talk up " to the rebellious organ or part, giving it orders just as one would a group of school boys or a squad of recruits in the army. Give the order positively and firmly, telling the organ just what you wish it to perform, repeating the command sharply several times. A tapping or mild slapping of the part, or the part of the body over the affected part, will act to attract the attention of the cell-group just as does the tapping of a man on the shoulder cause him to stop, turn around and listen to what you have to say. Now, please do not suppose that we are trying to tell you that the cells have ears and understand the words of the particular language you may be using. What really happens is that the sharply spoken words help you to form the mental image expressed by the words, and this meaning goes right to the spot, over the channels of the sympathetic nervous system operated by the Instinctive Mind, and is readily understood by the cell-groups, and even by the individual cells. As we have already said, an additional supply of Prana and the increased supply of blood also go to the affected region, being directed there by the concentrated attention of the person sending the command. The commands of a healer may be given in the same way, the Instinctive Mind of the patient taking up the command and forwarding it to the scene of the cell rebellion. This may seem almost childish to many of our students, but there are good scientific reasons behind it, and the Yogis consider it the simplest plan whereby mental commands may reach the cells. So do not discard it as worthless until you have tried it awhile. It has stood the test of centuries, and nothing better has been found to do the work.

If you wish to try this plan upon some portion of your body, or the body of someone else which is not functioning properly, gently slap the part with the flat palm of the hand, saying to it sharply (for instance) : " Here, Liver, you must do your work better—you are too sluggish to suit me—I expect you to do better from now on—get to work—get to work, I say, and stop this foolishness." These exact words are not necessary ; use any words which may come to you, so long as they convey a sharp positive command that the organ shall do its work. The heart's action may be improved in the same way, but one must proceed in a far more gentle manner, as the cell-group of the heart is possessed of a much higher degree of intelligence than that of the liver, for instance, and must be approached in a more respectful manner. Gently remind the heart that you expect it to do its work in a better manner, but speak to it politely and do not attempt to " bulldoze " it as you would the liver. The heart cell-group is the most intelligent of the groups controlling any of the organs—the liver group is the most stupid and less intelligent, being of a decidedly mulish disposition, whereas the heart is like a thoroughbred horse, intelligent and alert. If your liver is rebellious you must go for it vigorously, remembering its mulish propensities. The stomach is fairly intelligent, although not as much so as the heart. The Colon is quite obedient, although patient and long suffering. One may give the Colon commands to evacuate its contents at a certain time every morning (naming the hour), and if you will trust it sufficiently to go to the stool at that particular hour—keep your engagement, in fact—you will find that the Colon will in a short time do as you wish it to. But remember that the poor Colon has been greatly abused and it may take a little time to regain its confidence. Irregular menstruation may be regulated, and normal habits acquired, in a few months by marking the proper date on the calendar and then each day giving oneself a gentle treatment along the lines above mentioned, telling the cell-groups controlling the function that it is now so many days before the expected time and that you wish them to get ready and do their work, so that when the time arrives everything will be normal. As you near the time, call the group's attention that the time is growing shorter and that it must attend to its business. Do not give the commands in a trifling manner but as if you really meant them—and you must mean them—and they will be obeyed. We have seen many cases of irregular menstruation relieved in this way in from one to three months. This may sound ridiculous to you, but all we can say is to try it for yourself. We have not space to point out the method to be employed for each complaint, but you will readily see just what organ or group controls the seat of the trouble from what we have said in other chapters, and then give it its orders. If you do not know what organ is causing the trouble, you at least know the region of the disturbance and may direct your commands to that part of the body. It is not necessary for you to know the name of the organ—just direct your commands to the spot and say to it: "Here, *You*, etc." This book is not intended as a treatise upon the cure of disease, its object being to point out the road to health by preventing disease, but these little hints at restoring normal functioning to organs which have been misbehaving may help you somewhat.

You will be surprised at the measure of control which you may gain over your body by following the above method and variations of the same. You will be able to relieve your headaches by directing the blood to flow downward; you will be able to warm your cold feet by ordering the blood to flow to them in increased quantities, the Prana, of course, going along also; you may equalize the circulation, thus stimulating the entire body; you may relieve tired portions of the body. In fact, there is no end of the things you may do along this line if you have but the patience to try. If you do not know just what commands to give you may say to the part, "Here, you, get better—I want this pain to leave—I want you to do better," or something similar. But all this requires practice and patience, of course. There is no royal road to its accomplishment.

CHAPTER XX

PRANIC ENERGY

The student will notice, as he reads the chapters of this book, that there is an esoteric and an exoteric side of Hatha Yoga. By "esoteric" we mean "designed for only the specially initiated; private" (Webster's Dictionary), and by "exoteric" we mean "external; public—opp. to esoteric" (Webster's Dictionary). The exoteric or public side of the subject consists in the theory of the obtaining of nourishment from the food—the irrigating and eliminating properties of water—the advantage of the rays of the sun in prompting growth and health—the benefit of exercise—the advantage of proper breathing—the benefit to be derived from fresh air, etc., etc. These theories are well known to the Western world, as well as to the Eastern; to the non-occultist as well as the occultist, and both recognize their truth and the benefits to be obtained by putting them into practice. But there is another side, quite familiar to the Orientals and to occultists generally, but unfamiliar to the Western world and not generally known among those who pay no attention to occult studies. This esoteric phase of the subject revolves around the subject of what the Orientals know as Prana. The latter, and all occultists, know that man obtains Prana as well as nourishment from his food—Prana as well as a cleansing effect from the water he drinks—Prana properly distributed as well as mere muscular development in physical exercise—Prana as well as heat from the rays of the sun—Prana as well as oxygen from the air he breathes—and so on. This subject of Prana is interwoven with the entire Hatha Yoga Philosophy, and must be seriously considered by its students. This being the case, we must consider the question, "What is Prana?"

We have explained the nature and uses of Prana in our little book, "The Science of Breath," and also in our "Yogi Philosophy and Oriental Occultism," more generally known as "The Yogi Lessons" (1904). And we dislike to fill the pages of this book with what may seem to be a repetition of that which has appeared in our other books. But in this instance, and a few others, we must reprint what we have already said, for many people who read this book may not have seen our other publications, and to omit any mention of "Prana" would be unfair. And, then, a work on Hatha Yoga without a description of Prana would be absurd. We will not take up much space in our description and will try to give only the gist of the subject.

Occultists in all ages and lands have always taught, usually secretly to a few followers, that there was to be found in the air, in water, in the food, in the sunlight, everywhere, a substance or principle from which all activity, energy, power and vitality were derived. They differed in their term and names for this force, as well as in the details of their theories, but the main principle is to be found in all occult teachings and philosophies, and has for centuries past been found among the teachings and practices of the Oriental Yogis. We have preferred to designate this vital principle by the name by which it is known among the Hindu teachers and students—gurus and chelas—and have used for this purpose the Sanscrit word "Prana," meaning "Absolute Energy."

Occult authorities teach that the principle which the Hindus term "Prana" is the universal principle of energy or force, and that all energy or force is derived from that principle, or, rather, is a particular form of manifestation of that principle. These theories do not concern us in the consideration of the subject matter of this work, and we will therefore confine ourselves to an understanding of prana as the principle of energy exhibited in all living things, which distinguishes them from a lifeless thing. We may consider it as the active principle of life—Vital Force, if you please. It is found in all forms of life, from the amœba to man—from the most elementary form of plant life to the highest form of animal life. Prana is all pervading. It is found in all things having life and as the occult philosophy teaches that life is in all things—in every atom—the apparent lifelessness of some things being only a lesser degree of manifestation, we may understand their teachings that prana is everywhere, in everything. Prana must not be confounded with the Ego—that bit of Divine Spirit in every soul, around which clusters matter and energy. Prana is merely a form of energy used by the Ego in its material manifestation. When the Ego leaves the body, the prana, being no longer under its control, responds only to the orders of the individual atoms, or groups of atoms, forming the body, and as the body disintegrates and is resolved to its original elements, each atom takes with it sufficient prana to enable it to form new combinations, the unused prana returning to the great universal store-house from which it came. With the Ego in control, cohesion exists and the atoms are held together by the Will of the Ego.

Prana is the name by which we designate a universal principle, which principle is the essence of all motion, force or energy, whether manifested in gravitation, electricity, the revolution of the planets, and all forms of life, from the highest to the lowest. It may be called the soul of Force and Energy in all their forms, and that principle which, operating in a certain way, causes that form of activity which accompanies Life.

This great principle is in all forms of matter, and yet it is not matter. It is in the air, but it is not the air nor one of its chemical constituents. It is in the food we eat, and yet it is not the same as the nourishing substances in the food. It is in the water we drink, and yet it is not one or more of the chemical substances which combining make water. It is in the sunlight, but yet it is not the heat or the light rays. It is the "energy" in all these things—the things acting merely as a carrier.

And man is able to extract it from the air, food, water, sunlight and turn it to good account in his own organism. But do not misunderstand us; we have no intention of claiming that Prana is in these things merely that it may be used by man. Far from it—Prana is in these things fulfilling the great law of Nature, and man's ability to extract a portion of it and use it is merely an incident. The force would exist though man were not.

This great principle is in all forms of matter, and yet it is not matter. It is in the air, but it is not the air nor one of its chemical constituents. Animal and plant life breathe it in with the air, and yet if the air contained it not they would die even though they might be filled with air. It is taken up by the system along with the oxygen, and yet is not the oxygen.

Prana is in the atmospheric air, but it is also elsewhere, and it penetrates where the air cannot reach. The oxygen in the air plays an important part in sustaining animal life, and the carbon plays a similar part with plant life, but Prana has its own distinct part to play in the manifestation of life, aside from the physiological functions.

We are constantly inhaling the air charged with prana, and are as constantly extracting the latter from the air and appropriating it to our uses. Prana is found in its freest state in the atmospheric air, which when fresh is fairly charged with it, and we draw it to us more easily from the air than from any other source. In ordinary breathing we absorb and extract a normal supply of prana, but by controlled and regulated breathing (generally known as Yogi breathing) we are enabled to extract a greater supply, which is stored away in the brain and nerve centres, to be used when necessary. We may store away prana, just as the storage battery stores away electricity. The many powers attributed to advanced occultists is due largely to their knowledge of this fact and their intelligent use of this stored-up energy. The Yogis know that by certain forms of breathing they establish certain relations with the supply of prana and may draw on the same for what they require. Not only do they strengthen all parts of their body in this way, but the brain itself may receive increased energy from the same source, and latent faculties be developed and psychic powers attained. One who has mastered the science of storing away prana, either consciously or unconsciously, often radiates vitality and strength, which is felt by those coming in contact with him, and such a person may impart this strength to others, and give them increased vitality and health. What is called "magnetic healing" is performed in this way, although many practitioners are not aware of the source of their power.

Western scientists have been dimly aware of this great principle with which the air is charged, but finding that they could find no chemical trace of it, or make it register on any of their instruments, they have generally treated the Oriental theory with disdain. They could not explain this principle, and so denied it. They seem, however, to recognize that the air in certain places possesses a greater amount of "something" and sick people are directed by their physicians to seek such places in hopes of regaining lost health.

The oxygen in the air is appropriated by the blood and is made use of by the circulatory system. The prana in the air is appropriated by the nervous system, and is used in its work. And as the oxygenated blood is carried to all parts of the system, building up and replenishing, so is the prana carried to all parts of the nervous system, adding strength and vitality. If we think of prana as being the active principle of what we call " vitality," we will be able to form a much clearer idea of what an important part it plays in our lives. Just as is the oxygen in the blood used up by the wants of the system, so the supply of prana taken up by the nervous system, is exhausted by our thinking, willing, acting, etc., and in consequence constant replenishing is necessary. Every thought, every act, every effort of the will, every motion of a muscle, uses up a certain amount of what we call nerve force, which is really a form of prana. To move a muscle the brain sends out an impulse over the nerves, and the muscle contracts, and so much prana is expended. When it is remembered that the greater portion of prana acquired by man comes to him from the air inhaled, the importance of proper breathing is readily understood.

It will be noticed that the Western scientific theories regarding the breath confine themselves to the effects of the absorption of oxygen, and its use through the circulatory system, while the Yogi theory also takes into consideration the absorption of Prana, and its manifestation through the channels of the Nervous System. Before proceeding further, it may be as well to take a hasty glance at the Nervous System.

The Nervous System of man is divided into two great systems, *viz.*, the Cerebro-Spinal System and the Sympathetic System. The Cerebro-Spinal

System consists of that part of the Nervous System contained within the cranial cavity and the spinal canal, *viz.*, the brain and the spinal cord, together with the nerves which branch off from the same. This system presides over the functions of animal life known as volition, sensation, etc. The Sympathetic System includes all that part of the Nervous System located principally in the thoracic, abdominal and pelvic cavities, and which is distributed to the internal organs. It has control over the involuntary processes, such as growth, nutrition, etc.

The Cerebro-Spinal System attends to all the seeing, hearing, tasting, smelling, feeling, etc. It sets things in motion ; it is used by the Ego to think —to manifest consciousness. It is the instrument with which the Ego communicates with the outside world. This system may be likened to a telephone system, with the brain as the central office, and the spinal column and nerves as cable and wires respectively.

The brain is a great mass of nerve tissue, and consists of three parts, *viz.*, the Cerebrum or brain power, which occupies the upper, front, middle and back portion of the skull ; the Cerebellum, or " little brain," which fills the lower and back portion of the skull ; and the Medulla Oblongata, which is the broadened commencement of the spinal cord, lying before and in front of the Cerebellum.

The Cerebrum is the organ of that part of the mind which manifests itself in intellectual action. The Cerebellum regulates the movements of the voluntary muscles. The Medulla Oblongata is the upper enlarged end of the spinal cord, and from it and the

Cerebrum branch forth the Cranial Nerves which reach to various parts of the head, to the organs of special sense, and to some of the thoracic and abdominal organs, and to the organs of respiration.

The Spinal Cord, or spinal marrow, fills the spinal canal in the vertebral column, or " backbone." It is a long mass of nerve tissue, branching off at the several vertebrae to nerves communicating with all parts of the body. The Spinal Cord is like a large telephone cable, and the emerging nerves are like the private wires connecting therewith.

The Sympathetic Nervous System consists of a double chain of Ganglia on the side of the spinal column, and scattered ganglia in the head, neck, chest and abdomen. (A ganglion is a mass of nervous matter including nerve cells.) These ganglia are connected with each other by filaments, and are also connected with the Cerebro-Spinal System by motor and sensory nerves. From these ganglia numerous fibres branch out to the organs of the body, blood-vessels, etc. At various points, the nerves meet together and form what are known as plexuses. The Sympathetic System practically controls the involuntary processes, such as circulation, respiration and digestion.

The power or force transmitted from the brain to all parts of the body by means of the nerves, is known to Western science as " nerve force," although the Yogi knows it to be a manifestation of Prana. In character and rapidity it resembles the electric current. It will be seen that without this " nerve force " the heart cannot beat ; the blood cannot circulate ; the lungs cannot breathe ; the various organs cannot function; in fact, the machinery of the body comes to a stop without it. Nay, more, even the brain cannot think without Prana be present. When these facts are considered, the importance of the absorption of Prana must be evident to all, and the Science of Breath assumes an importance even greater than that accorded it by Western science.

The Yogi teachings go further than does Western science, in one important feature of the Nervous System. We allude to what Western science terms the "Solar Plexus," and which it considers as merely one of a series of certain matted nets of sympathetic nerves with their ganglia found in various parts of the body. Yogi science teaches that this Solar Plexus is really a most important part of the Nervous System, and that it is a form of brain, playing one of the principal parts in the human economy. Western science seems to be moving gradually towards a recognition of this fact which has been known to the Yogis of the East for centuries, and some recent Western writers have termed the Solar Plexus the "Abdominal Brain." The Solar Plexus is situated in the Epigastric region, just back of the "pit of the stomach" on either side of the spinal column. It is composed of white and gray brain matter, similar to that composing the other brains of man. It has control of the main internal organs of man, and plays a much more important part than is generally recognized. We will not go into the Yogi theory regarding the Solar Plexus, further than to say that they know it as the great central store-house of Prana. Men have been known to be instantly killed by a severe blow over the Solar Plexus, and prize-fighters recognize its vulnerability and frequently temporarily paralyze their opponents by a blow over this region.

The name "Solar" is well bestowed on this "brain," as it radiates strength and energy to all parts of the body, even the upper brains depending largely upon it as a store-house of Prana. Sooner or later Western science will fully recognize the real function of the Solar Plexus, and will accord to it a far more important place than it now occupies in their text-books and teachings.

CHAPTER XXI

PRANIC EXERCISES

We have told you in other chapters of this book, how Prana may be obtained from the air, food and water. We have given you detailed instruction in breathing, in eating, in the use of fluids. There remains but little more for us to say upon the subject. But before leaving it, we have thought it well to give you a bit of the higher theory and practice of Hatha Yoga, touching upon the acquirement and distribution of Prana. We allude to what has been called "Rhythmic Breathing," which is the keynote to much of the Hatha Yoga practices.

All is in vibration. From the tiniest atom to the greatest sun, everything is in a state of vibration. There is nothing in absolute rest in nature. A single atom deprived of vibration would wreck the universe. In incessant vibration the universal work is performed. Matter is being constantly played upon by energy and countless forms and numberless varieties result, and yet even the forms and varieties are not permanent. They begin to change the moment they are created, and from them are born innumerable forms, which in turn change, and give rise to newer forms, and so on and on, in infinite succession. Nothing is permanent in the world of forms, and yet the great Reality is unchangeable. Forms are but appearances—they come, they go, but the Reality is eternal and unchangeable.

The atoms of the human body are in constant vibration. Unceasing changes are occurring. In a few months there is almost a complete change in the matter composing the body, and scarcely a single atom now composing your body will be found in it a few months hence. Vibration, constant vibration. Change, constant change.

In all vibration is to be found a certain rhythm. Rhythm pervades the universe. The swing of the planets around the sun; the rise and fall of the sea; the beating of the heart; the ebb and flow of the tide; all follow rhythmic laws. The rays of the sun reach us; the rain descends upon us, in obedience to the same law. All growth is but an exhibition of this law. All motion is a manifestation of the law of rhythm.

Our bodies are as much subject to rhythmic laws as is the planet in its revolution around the sun. Much of the esoteric side of the Yogi Science of Breath is based upon this known principle of nature. By falling in with the rhythm of the body, the Yogi manages to absorb a great amount of Prana, which he disposes of to bring about results desired by him. We will speak of this at greater length later on.

The body which you occupy is like a small inlet running in to the land from the sea. Although apparently subject only to its own laws, it is really subject to the ebb and flow of the tides of the ocean. The great sea of life is swelling and receding, rising and falling, and we are responding to its vibrations and rhythm. In a normal condition we receive the vibration and rhythm of the great ocean of life, and respond to it, but at times the mouth of the inlets seems choked up with débris, and we fail to receive the impulse from Mother Ocean, and inharmony manifests within us.

You have heard how a note on a violin, if sounded repeatedly and in rhythm, will start into motion vibrations which will in time destroy a bridge. The same result is true when a regiment of soldiers crosses a bridge, the order being always given to "break step" on such an occasion, lest the vibration bring down both bridge and regiment. These manifestations of the effect of rhythmic motion will give you an idea of the effect on the body of rhythmic breathing. The whole system catches the vibration and becomes in harmony with the will, which causes the rhythmic motion of the lungs, and while in such complete harmony will respond readily to orders from the will. With the body thus attuned, the Yogi finds no difficulty in increasing the circulation in any part of the body by an order from the will, and in the same way he can direct an increased current of nerve force to any part or organ, strengthening and stimulating it.

In the same way the Yogi by rhythmic breathing "catches the swing," as it were, and is able to absorb and control a greatly increased amount of prana, which is then at the disposal of his will. He can and does use it as a vehicle for sending forth thoughts to others and for attracting to him all those whose thoughts are keyed in the same vibration. The phenomena of telepathy, thought transference, mental healing, mesmerism, etc., which subjects are creating such an interest in the Western world at the present time, but which have been known to the

Yogis for centuries, can be greatly increased and augmented if the person sending forth the thoughts will do so after rhythmic breathing. Rhythmic breathing will increase the value of mental healing, magnetic healing, etc., several hundred per cent.

In rhythmic breathing the main thing to be acquired is the mental idea of rhythm. To those who know anything of music, the idea of measured counting is familiar. To others, the rhythmic step of the soldier : "Left, right ; left, right ; left, right ; one, two, three, four ; one, two, three, four," will convey the idea.

The Yogi bases his rhythmic time upon a unit corresponding with the beat of his heart. The heart beat varies in different persons, but the heart beat unit of each person is the proper rhythmic standard for that particular individual in his rhythmic breathing. Ascertain your normal heart beat, by placing your fingers over your pulse, and then count : "1, 2, 3, 4, 5, 6 ; 1, 2, 3, 4, 5, 6," etc., until the rhythm becomes firmly fixed in your mind. A little practice will fix the rhythm, so that you will be able to easily reproduce it. The beginner usually inhales in about six pulse units, but he will be able to greatly increase this by practice.

The Yogi rule for rhythmic breathing is that the units of inhalation and exhalation should be the same, while the units for retention and between breaths should be one-half the number of those of inhalation and exhalation.

The following exercise in Rhythmic Breathing should be thoroughly mastered, as it forms the basis of numerous other exercises, to which reference will be made later.

(1) Sit erect, in an easy posture, being sure to hold the chest, neck and head as nearly in a straight line as possible, with shoulders slightly thrown back and hands resting easily on the lap. In this position the weight of the body is largely supported by the ribs, and the position may be easily maintained. The Yogi has found that one cannot get the best effect of rhythmic breathing with the chest drawn in and the abdomen protruding.

(2) Inhale slowly a Complete Breath, counting six pulse units.

(3) Retain, counting three pulse units.

(4) Exhale slowly through the nostrils, counting six pulse units.

(5) Count three pulse beats between breaths.

(6) Repeat a number of times, but avoid fatiguing yourself at the start.

(7) When you are ready to close the exercise, practise the Cleansing Breath, which will rest you and cleanse the lungs.

After a little practice you will be able to increase the duration of the inhalations and exhalations, until about fifteen pulse units are consumed. In this increase, remember that the units for retention and between breaths is one-half the units for inhalation and exhalation.

Do not overdo yourself in your effort to increase the duration of the breath, but pay as much attention as possible to acquiring the "rhythm," as that is more important than the length of the breath. Practise and try until you get the measured "swing" of the movement, and until you can almost "feel" the rhythm of the vibratory motion throughout your whole body. It will require a little practice and perseverance, but your pleasure at your improvement will make the task an easy one. The Yogi is a most patient and persevering man, and his great attainments are due largely to the possession of these qualities.

Prana Generating

Lying flat on the floor or bed, completely relaxed, with hands resting lightly over the Solar Plexus (over the pit of the stomach, where the ribs begin to separate), breathe rhythmically. After the rhythm is fully established *will* that each inhalation shall draw in an increased supply of prana or vital energy from the Universal supply, which will be taken up by the nervous system and stored in the Solar Plexus. At each exhalation will that the prana or vital energy shall be distributed all over the body, to every organ and part; to every muscle, cell and atom; to nerve, artery and vein; from the top of your head to the soles of your feet; invigorating, strengthening and stimulating every nerve; recharging every nerve centre; sending energy, force and strength all over the system. While exercising the will, try to form a mental picture of the inrushing prana, coming in through the lungs and being taken up at once by the Solar Plexus, then with the exhaling effort, being sent to all parts of the system, down to the finger tips and down to the toes. It is not necessary to use the Will with an effort. Simply commanding that which you wish to produce and then making the mental picture of it is all that is necessary. Calm command with the mental picture is far better than forcible willing, which only dissipates force needlessly. The above exercise is most helpful and greatly refreshes and strengthens the nervous system and produces a restful feeling all over the body. It is especially beneficial in cases where one is tired or feels a lack of energy.

Changing the Circulation

Lying down or sitting erect, breathe rhythmically, and with the exhalations direct the circulation to any part you wish, which may be suffering from imperfect circulation. This is effective in cases of cold feet or in cases of headache, the blood being sent downward in both cases, in the first case warming the feet, and in the latter relieving the brain from too great pressure. You will often feel a warm feeling in the legs as the circulation moves downward. The circulation is largely under the control of the will and rhythmic breathing renders the task easier.

Recharging

If you feel that your vital energy is at a low ebb, and that you need to store up a new supply quickly, the best plan is to place the feet close together (side by side, of course) and to lock the fingers of both hands in any way that seems the most comfortable. This closes the circuit, as it were, and prevents any escape of prana through the extremities. Then breathe rhythmically a few times, and you will feel the effect of the recharging.

Brain Stimulation

The Yogis have found the following exercise most useful in stimulating the action of the brain for the purpose of producing clear thinking and reasoning. It has a wonderful effect in clearing the brain and nervous system, and those engaged in mental work will find it most useful to them, both in the direction of enabling them to do better work and also as a means of refreshing the mind and clearing it after arduous mental labour.

Sit in an erect posture, keeping the spinal column straight, and the eyes well to the front, letting the hands rest on the upper part of the legs. Breathe rhythmically, but instead of breathing through both nostrils, as in the ordinary exercises, press the left nostril close with the thumb, and inhale through the right nostril. Then remove the thumb, and close the right nostril with the finger, and then exhale through the left nostril. Then, without changing the fingers, inhale through the left nostril, and changing fingers, exhale through the right. Then inhale through right and exhale through left, and so on, alternating nostrils as above mentioned, closing the unused nostril with the thumb or forefinger. This is one of the oldest forms of Yogi breathing, and is quite important and valuable, and is well worthy of acquirement. But it is quite amusing to the Yogis to know that to the Western world this method is often held out as being the " whole secret " of Yogi Breathing. To the minds of many Western readers, " Yogi Breathing " suggests nothing more than a picture of a Hindu, sitting erect, and alternating nostrils in the act of breathing. "Only this and nothing more." We trust that this little work will open the eyes of the Western world to the great possibilities of Yogi Breathing, and the numerous methods whereby it may be employed.

Yogi Grand Psychic Breath

The Yogis have a favourite form of psychic breathing which they practise occasionally, to which has been given a Sanscrit term of which the above is a general equivalent. We have given it last, as it requires practice on the part of the student in the line of rhythmic breathing and mental imagery, which he has now acquired by means of the preceding exercises. The general principles of the Grand Breath may be summed up in the old Hindu saying, "Blessed is the Yogi who can breathe through his bones." This exercise will fill the entire system with prana, and the student will emerge from it with every bone, muscle, nerve, cell, tissue, organ and part energized and attuned by the prana and the rhythm of the breath. It is a general house-cleaning of the system, and he who practises it carefully will feel as if he had been given a new body, freshly created, from the crown of his head to the tips of his toes. We will let the exercise speak for itself.

(1) Lie in a relaxed position, at perfect ease.

(2) Breathe rhythmically until the rhythm is perfectly established.

(3) Then, inhaling and exhaling, form the mental image of the breath being drawn up through the bones of the legs, and then forced out through them ;

then through the bones of the arms ; then through the top of the skull ; then through the stomach ; then through the reproductive region ; then as if it were travelling upward and downward along the spinal column ; and then as if the breath were being inhaled and exhaled through every pore of the skin, the whole body being filled with prana and life.

(4) Then (breathing rhythmically) send the current of prana to the Seven Vital Centres, in turn, as follows, using the mental picture as in previous exercises :

(*a*) To the forehead.
(*b*) To the back of the head.
(*c*) To the base of the brain.
(*d*) To the Solar Plexus.
(*e*) To the Sacral Region (lower part of the spine).
(*f*) To the region of the navel.
(*g*) To the reproductive region.

Finish by sweeping the current of prana, to and fro, from head to feet, several times.

(5) Finish with Cleansing Breath.

CHAPTER XXII

THE SCIENCE OF RELAXATION

THE Science of Relaxation forms a very important part of the Hatha Yoga philosophy and many of the Yogis have devoted much care and study to this branch of the subject. At first glance it may appear to the average reader that the idea of teaching people how to relax—how to rest—is ridiculous, as everyone should know how to perform this simple feat. And the average man is right—in part. Nature teaches us how to relax and rest to perfection—the infant is a past-master in the science. But as we have grown older we have acquired many artificial habits and have allowed Nature's original habits to lapse. And so at the present time the people of the Western world may well accept from the Yogis a little teaching along the lines of this subject.

The average physician could give some very interesting testimony on the subject of the failure of the people to understand the first principles of relaxation—he knows that a large percentage of the nervous troubles of the people are due to ignorance of the subject of "rest."

Rest and relaxation are very different things from "loafing," "laziness," etc. On the contrary, those who have mastered the science of relaxation are usually the most active and energetic kind of people, but they waste no energy; with them every motion counts.

Let us consider the question of relaxation and try to see just what it means. In order to better comprehend it let us first consider its opposite—contraction. When we wish to contract a muscle, in order that we may perform some action, we send an impulse from the brain to the muscle, an extra supply of Prana being conveyed to it, and the muscle contracts. The Prana travels over the motor nerves, reaches the muscle and causes it to draw its ends together and to thus exert a pull upon the limb or part which we wish to move, bringing it into action. If we wish to dip our pen into the inkwell, our desire manifests into action by our brain sending a current of Prana to certain muscles in our right arm, hand and fingers, and the muscles, contracting in turn, carry our pen to the inkwell, dip it in, and bring it back to our paper. And so with every act of the body, conscious or unconscious. In the conscious act the conscious faculties send a message to the Instinctive Mind, which immediately obeys the order by sending the current of Prana to the desired part. In the unconscious movement the Instinctive Mind does not wait for orders, but attends to the whole work itself, both the ordering and the executing. But every action, conscious or unconscious, uses up a certain amount of Prana, and if the amount so used is in excess of the amount which the system has been in the habit of storing the result is that one becomes weakened and generally "used up." The fatigue of a particular muscle is somewhat different, and results from the unaccustomed work it has been called upon to perform, because of the unusual amount of Prana which has been directed toward contracting it.

We have spoken so far only of the actual movements of the body, resulting from muscular contraction, proceeding from the current of prana directed to the muscle. There is another form of the using up of prana and the consequent wear and tear upon the muscles, which is not so familiar to the minds of most of us. Those of our students who live in the cities will recognize our meaning when we compare the waste of prana to the waste of water occasioned by the failure to turn off the faucet in the washbowl and the resulting trickling away of the water hour after hour. Well, this is just what many of us are doing all the time—we are allowing our prana to trickle away in a constant stream, with a consequent wear and tear upon our muscles, and, indeed, upon the whole system, from the brain down.

Our students are doubtless familiar with the axiom of psychology, "Thought takes form in action." Our first impulse when we wish to do a thing is to make the muscular movement necessary to the accomplishment of the action proceeding from the thought. But we may be restrained from making the movement by another thought, which shows us the desirability of repressing the action. We may be inflamed with anger and may experience a desire to strike the person causing the anger. The thought is scarcely formed in our mind before the first steps toward striking are taken. But before the muscle fairly moves our better judgment causes us to send a repressing impulse (all this in the fraction of a second), and the opposite set of muscles holds back the action of the first set. The double action, ordering and countermanding, is performed so quickly that the mind cannot grasp any sense of motion, but nevertheless the muscle had begun to quiver with the striking impulse by the time the restraining impulse operated the opposing set of muscles and held back the movement.

This same principle, carried to still further refinements, causes a slight current of prana to the muscle, and a consequent slight muscular contraction, to follow many unrestrained thoughts, with a constant waste of prana and a perpetual wear and tear upon the nervous system and muscles. Many people of an excitable, irritable, emotional habit of mind constantly keep their nerves in action and their muscles tense by unrestrained and uncontrolled mental states. Thoughts take form in action, and a person of the temperament and habits just described is constantly allowing his thoughts to manifest in the currents sent to the muscles and the countermanding current immediately following. On the contrary, the person who has naturally, or has cultivated, a calm, controlled mind, will have no such impulses with their accompanying results. He moves along well poised and well in hand, and does not allow his thoughts to run away with him. He is a Master, not a slave.

The custom of this attempt of the excitable thoughts to take form in action, and their repressing often grows into a regular habit—becomes chronic—and the nerves and muscles of the person so afflicted are constantly under a strain, the result being that there is a constant drain upon the vitality, or prana, of the entire system. Such people usually have a number of their muscles in a tense condition, which means that a constant, though not necessarily strong, current of prana is being poured out to them, and the nerves are constantly in use carrying the prana. We remember hearing the story of the good old woman who was taking a ride on the railroad to a nearby town. So rare was the pleasure to her and so anxious was she to get to her destination that she could not settle herself back into her seat, but, on the contrary, sat on the edge of the seat, with her body well bent forward, during the whole sixteen miles of the journey; she was mentally trying to help the train along by giving it a mental urge in the right direction. This old lady's thoughts were fixed so firmly upon her journey's end that the thought took form in action and caused a muscular contraction in place of the relaxation which she should have indulged in during the trip. Many of us are just as bad; we strain forward anxiously, if we happen to be looking at an object, and in one way or another we tense a number of our muscles all the time. We clench our fists, or frown, or close our lips tight, or bite our lips, or set our jaws together, or something else along the same line of expressing our mental states in physical action. All this is waste. And so are the bad habits of beating the "devil's tattoo" on the table or arms of the chair, twirling the thumbs, wiggling the fingers, tapping on the floor with our toes, chewing gum, whittling sticks, biting lead pencils, and, last but not least, rocking nervously to and fro on a rocking chair. All these things, and many others too numerous to mention, are waste, pure waste.

Now that we understand something about muscular

contraction let us again take up the subject of the Science of Relaxation.

In relaxation there is practically no current of prana being poured out. (There is always a small amount sent to the different parts of the body, in health, in order to maintain a normal condition, but this is a very small current compared to that sent out to contract a muscle.) In relaxation the muscles and nerves are at rest, and the prana is being stored up and conserved, instead of being dissipated in reckless expenditures.

Relaxation may be observed in young children, and among the animals. Some adults have it, and, mark you this, such individuals are always noted for their endurance, strength, vigour and vitality. The lazy tramp is not an instance of relaxation; there is a great difference between relaxation and "loaf." The former is a sensible rest between working efforts, the result being that the work is done better and with less effort—the latter is the result of a mental indisposition to work and the consequent action (or inaction) resulting from such thought taking form.

The person understanding Relaxation and the conserving of energy accomplishes the best work. He uses a pound of effort to do the pound of work, and does not waste, slop over, or allow his strength to trickle away. The average person not understanding the law uses up from three to twenty-five times the energy needed to do his work, be that work mental or physical. If you doubt this statement watch the people with whom you come in contact and see how many waste motions they make and how many exaggerated movements, etc., they manifest. They haven't themselves well in hand mentally, and the result is physical prodigality.

In the Orient, where the Yogi gurus, or teachers, have classes of chelas, or students, who receive their instruction not from books, but from the words of the teacher, many object lessons from nature and illustrations are given in order that the idea may be associated in the mind of the student, with some material object or living thing. The Hatha Yoga gurus, when teaching the lesson of Relaxation, often direct their student's attention to the cat, or animals of the cat-tribe, the panther or leopard being a favourite illustration in lands where these animals are found.

Did you ever notice a cat in repose, resting? And have you ever watched a cat crouching before a mouse-hole? In the latter case do you recall how the cat crouched in an easy, graceful attitude—no muscular contraction, no tense attitude; a beautiful picture of intense vitality in repose, but ready for instant action. Still and motionless remains the animal; to all appearances it might be asleep or dead. But wait till it moves! Then like a flash of lightning it darts forward. The repose of the waiting cat, although absolutely devoid of movement or tense muscles, is a very live repose—a very different thing from "laziness." And note the entire absence of quivering muscles; of nerves "on edge"; of beaded perspiration. The machinery of action is not strained with waiting. There is no waste motion or tension; all is in readiness, and when the moment of action comes the prana is hurled into fresh muscles and untired nerves and the action follows the thought like the spark from the electric machine.

The Hatha Yogis do well to use the cat family as an illustration of grace, vitality and repose

In fact, there can be no great power of quick and effective action unless the ability to relax is also there. People who fidget, fret, and fume, and "stamp" up and down, are not the people who do the best work; they wear themselves out before the hour for action arrives. The man who may be depended upon is the one who possesses calmness, the ability to relax, repose. But let not the "fidgety" person despair; relaxation and repose may be cultivated and acquired just as may be other desirable "gifts."

In our next chapter we will give a few simple instructions to those wishing to acquire a working knowledge of the Science of Relaxation.

CHAPTER XXIII

RULES FOR RELAXATION

THOUGHTS take form in action, and actions react upon the mind. These two truths stand together. One is as true as the other. We have heard much of the influence of the mind over the body, but we must not forget that the body, or its attitudes and positions, react upon the mind and influence mental states. We must remember these two truths in considering the question of relaxation.

Much of the harmful and foolish practices and habits of muscular contraction are caused by mental states taking form in physical action. And, on the other hand, many of our mental states have been produced or encouraged by habits of physical carelessness, etc. When we are angry the emotion is apt to manifest in our clenching the fist. And, on the other hand, if we cultivate the habit of clenching the fists, frowning, drawing together the lips and assuming a scowl, we will be very apt to get the mind into such a condition that the least thing will plunge it into a spell of anger. You all know of the experiment of forcing a smile to the lips and eyes and maintaining it for a while, which generally results in making you *feel* " smiling " after a few minutes.

One of the first steps toward preventing the harmful practices of muscular contraction, with its resulting waste of prana and wearing out of the nerves, is to cultivate a mental attitude of calm and repose. This may be done, but it will be hard work at first; but you will be well repaid for your trouble in the end. Mental poise and repose may be brought about by the eradication of Worry and Anger. Of course, Fear really underlies both Worry and Anger, but as we are perhaps more familiar with the idea of Worry and Anger as being elementary mental states, we will so treat them. The Yogi trains himself from youth to eradicate or inhibit both of these emotions, and the result is that after he has developed his full powers he is absolutely serene and calm and presents the appearance of power and strength. He creates the same impression that is conveyed by the mountain, the sea, or other manifestations of restrained force. One in his presence feels that here is indeed great strength and power in perfect repose. The Yogi considers Anger an unworthy emotion, natural in the lower animals and in savage man, but totally out of place in the developed man. He considers it a sort of temporary insanity and pities the man who loses his self-control sufficiently to fly into a rage. He knows that nothing is accomplished by it, and that it is a useless waste of energy and a positive injury to the brain and nervous system, besides being a weakening element in one's moral nature and spiritual growth. This does not mean that the Yogi is a timid creature without any "backbone." On the contrary, he does not know the existence of Fear, and his calmness is instinctively felt to be the indication of strength, not weakness. Have you ever noticed that the men of the greatest strength are almost invariably free from bluster and threats? They leave that for those who are weak and wish to be thought strong. The Yogi also has eradicated Worry from his mental condition. He has learned to know that it is a foolish waste of energy, which results in no good and always works harm. He believes in earnest thought when problems have to be solved, obstacles surmounted, but he never descends to Worry. He regards Worry as waste energy and motion, and also as being unworthy of a developed man. He knows his own nature and powers too well to allow himself to worry. He has gradually emancipated himself from its curse and teaches his students that the freeing of oneself from Anger and Worry is the first step in practical Yoga.

While the controlling of the unworthy emotions of the lower nature really form a part of other branches of the Yogi Philosophy, it has a direct bearing upon the question of Relaxation, inasmuch as it is a fact that one habitually free from Anger and Worry is correspondingly free from the principal causes of involuntary muscular contraction and nerve-waste. The man possessed by Anger has muscles on the strain from chronic involuntary impulses from the brain. The man who is wrapped in the folds of Worry is constantly in a state of nervous strain and muscular contraction So it will readily be seen that when one cuts himself loose from these weakening emotions he at the same time frees himself from the greater part of the muscular contraction, of which we have spoken. If you would be free from this great source of waste, manage to get rid of the emotions causing it.

And, on the other hand, the practice of relaxing—of avoiding the tense condition of the muscles, in everyday life—will react upon the mind, and will enable it to regain its normal poise and repose. It is a rule that works both ways.

One of the first lessons in physical relaxation the Hatha Yogis give to their pupils is given in the next paragraph. Before beginning, however, we wish to impress upon the mind of the student the keynote of the Yogi practice of Relaxation. It consists of two words: "LET GO." If you master the meaning of these two words and are able to put them into practice you have grasped the secret of the Yogi theory and practice of Relaxation.

The following is a favourite Yogi exercise in Relaxation: Lie down flat on the back. Relax as thoroughly as you can, letting go of all the muscles. Then, still relaxed, let your mind wander over the body from the head down to the toes. In doing this you will find that here and there are certain muscles still in a tense condition—let go of them. If you do this thoroughly (you will improve by practice) you will end by having every muscle in the body fully relaxed and the nerves at rest. Take a few deep breaths, lying quietly and fully relaxed. You may vary this exercise by gently rolling over to one side, and again relaxing completely. Then roll over to the other side and relax completely. This is not as easy as it appears at first reading, as you will realize from a few trials. But do not be discouraged. Try it again until you master the "knack." While lying relaxed carry in your mind that you are lying on a soft, downy couch and that your body and limbs are as heavy as lead. Repeat the words several times, slowly: "Heavy as lead, heavy as lead," at the same time lifting the arms and then withdrawing the prana from them by ceasing to contract the muscles, and allowing them to drop of their own weight to the sides. This is a hard thing for most persons to do at first trial. They are unable to let their arms drop of their own weight, so firmly has the habit of involuntary muscular contraction fastened itself upon them. After you have mastered the arms try the legs, one at a time, then both together. Let them drop of their own weight and remain perfectly relaxed. Rest between trials and do not be strenuous in the exercise, as the idea is to rest yourself, as well as to acquire the control over the muscles. Then lift the head and allow it to drop in the same way. Then lie still and form the mental image of the couch, or floor, bearing the entire weight of the body. You may laugh at this idea, believing that when you lie down you always let the couch bear all of your weight, but you are mistaken. You will find that, in spite of yourself, you are endeavouring to support a part of your weight by tensing some of the muscles—you are trying to hold yourself up. Stop this and let the couch attend to this work for you. You are as foolish as was the old woman who sat on the edge of the car-seat and tried to help the train along. Take the sleeping child for your model. It allows its entire weight to rest on the bed. If you doubt this, look at the bed upon which a child has been sleeping and see the "dents" in it—the impress of its little body. If you find it difficult to catch the knack of this complete relaxation it may help you to carry the mental image of being as "limp" as a wet cloth—limp all over from head to foot—lying loose and limp, without a trace of stiffness. A little practice will soon work wonders with you, and you will arise from this "resting exercise" much refreshed and feeling able to do your work well.

There are also a number of other exercises in Relaxation taught and practised by the Hatha Yogis, the following being among the best of what are known to the Yogis by the term (free translation) "Loosen-up" exercises:

A Few "Loosen-up" Exercises

(1) Withdraw all prana from the hand, letting the muscles relax so that the hand will swing loosely from the wrist, apparently lifeless. Shake it backward and forward from the wrist. Then try the other hand the same way. Then both hands together. A little practice will give you the correct idea.

(2) This is more difficult than the first exercise. It consists in making the fingers limp and relaxed and swinging them loosely from the knuckles. Try first one hand and then the other, then both.

(3) Withdraw all prana from the arms and let them hang limp and loose by the sides. Then swing the body from side to side, letting the arms swing (like empty coat-sleeves) from the motion of the body, making no effort of the arms themselves. First one arm and then the other, and then both. This exercise may be varied by twisting the body around in various ways, letting the arms swing

loose. You will get the idea if you will think of loose coat-sleeves.

(4) Relax the forearm, letting it swing loose from the elbow. Impart a motion from the upper-arm, but avoid contracting the muscles of the forearm. Shake the forearm around limp and loose. First one arm, then the other, then both.

(5) Let the foot be completely relaxed and swung loose from the ankle. This will require some little practice, as the muscles moving the foot are generally in a more or less contracted condition. But baby's foot is loose enough when he is not using it. First one foot, then the other.

(6) Relax the leg, withdrawing all prana from it and letting it swing loose and limp from the knee. Then swing it and shake it. First one leg and then the other.

(7) Stand on a cushion, stool or large book and let one leg swing loose and limp from the thigh, after having relaxed it completely. First one leg and then the other.

(8) Raise the arms straight above the head, and then, withdrawing all prana from them, let them drop of their own weight to the sides.

(9) Lift the knee up in front as high as you can and then draw all prana from it and let it drop back of its own weight.

(10) Relax the head, letting it drop forward, and then swing it about by the motion of the body. Then, sitting back in a chair, relax it and let it drop backward. It will, of course, drop in any direction the moment you withdraw the prana from it. To get the right idea, think of a person falling asleep,

who, the moment sleep overpowers him, relaxes and stops contracting the muscles of the neck, allowing the head to drop forward.

(11) Relax the muscles of the shoulders and chest, allowing the upper part of the chest to fall forward loose and limp.

(12) Sit in a chair and relax the muscles of the waist, which will allow the upper part of the body to pitch forward like that of a child who falls asleep in its chair and gradually falls out.

(13) One who has mastered these exercises so far may, if he sees fit, relax his whole body, commencing with the neck, until he gets down to the knees, when he will drop gently to the floor "all in a heap." This is a valuable acquirement, as in case of one slipping or falling by accident. The practice of this entire body relaxation will do much to protect them from injury. You will notice that a young child will relax in this way when it falls, and is scarcely affected by severe falls which would seriously bruise adults, or even break their limbs. The same phenomenon may be noticed in the cases of intoxicated persons who have lost control of the muscles and are in an almost complete state of relaxation. When they fall they come down "all in a heap" and suffer comparatively little injury.

In practising these exercises repeat each of them several times and then pass on to the next one. These exercises may be almost indefinitely extended and varied, according to the ingenuity and power of invention of the student. Make your own exercises, if you will, using the above as suggestions.

Practising relaxation exercises gives one a

consciousness of self-control and repose, which is valuable. *Strength in repose* is the idea to be carried in the mind when thinking of the Yogi Relaxation theories. It is useful in quieting overwrought nerves ; is an antidote for what is known as " muscle-bound " conditions resulting from the employment of certain sets of muscles in one's daily work or exercise, and is a valuable acquirement in the direction of allowing one to rest himself at will and to thus regain his vitality in the shortest possible time. The Oriental people understand the science of relaxation and employ it in their daily life. They will undertake journeys which would frighten a Western man, and after travelling many miles will make a resting place upon which they will throw themselves down, relaxing every muscle and with-drawing the prana from all the voluntary muscles, allowing themselves to remain limp and apparently lifeless from head to foot. They indulge in a doze at the same time, if practicable, but if not they remain wide awake, with senses active and alert, but with the bodily muscles as above stated. One hour of this rest refreshes them as much, or more, than a night's sleep does the average man. They start on their journey again, refreshed and with new life and energy. Nearly all the wandering races and tribes have acquired this knowledge. It seems to have been intuitively acquired by the American Indian, the Arab, the savage tribes of Africa, and, in fact, races in all parts of the world. Civilized man has allowed this gift to lapse, because he has ceased to make the long journeys on foot, but it would be well for him to regain this lost knowledge and to use same to relieve the fatigue and nerve-exhaustion of the strenuous business life, which has taken the place of the old wandering life, with all its hardships.

Stretching

"Stretching" is another method of resting employed by the Yogis. At first sight this will seem to be the reverse of relaxation, but it is really akin to it, inasmuch as it withdraws the tension from the muscles which have been habitually contracted, and sends the prana through them to all parts of the system, equalizing pranic conditions to the benefit of all the parts of the body. Nature impels us to yawn and stretch when we are fatigued. Let us take a lesson from her book. Let us learn to stretch at will as well as involuntarily. This is not so easy as you may imagine and you will have to practise somewhat before you get the full benefit from it.

Take up the Relaxation exercises in the order in which they are given in this chapter, but instead of relaxing each part in turn simply stretch them. Begin with the feet, and then work up to the legs, and then up to the arms and head. Stretch in all sorts of ways, twisting your legs, feet, arms, hands, head and body around in a way you feel like to get the full benefit of the stretch. Don't be afraid of yawning, either; that is simply one form of stretch. In stretching you will, of course, tense and contract muscles, but the rest and relief comes in the subsequent relaxation of them. Carry in your mind the "let-go" idea, rather than that of muscular exertion. We cannot attempt to give exercises in stretching, as the variety open to the student is so great that he should not require to have illustrations given him. Just let him give way to the mental idea of a good, restful stretch, and Nature will tell him what to do. Here is one general suggestion, however : Stand on the floor, with your legs spread apart and your arms extended over your head, also spread apart. Then raise yourself on your toes and stretch yourself out gradually, as if you were trying to reach the ceiling. A most simple exercise, but wonderfully refreshing.

A variation of stretching may be effected by "shaking" yourself around loose and limp, employing as many parts of your body as you can. The Newfoundland dog, shaking the water from his skin when he emerges from the water, will give you a general idea of what we mean.

All of these plans of relaxing, if properly entered into and carried out, will leave the one practising them with a sense of renewed energy and an inclination to again resume work, the same feeling as one experiences after arising from a healthy sleep and a subsequent good rub-down in the bath.

Mental Relaxation Exercise

Perhaps it will be as well for us to give an exercise in Mental Relaxation before we conclude this chapter. Of course, physical relaxation reacts on the mind and rests it. But Mental Relaxation also reacts upon the body and rests it. So this exercise may reach the needs of some who have not found just what they required in the preceding pages of this chapter.

Sit quietly in a relaxed and easy position and

withdraw the mind as far as possible from outside objects and from thoughts which require active mental effort. Let your thought reach inward and dwell upon the real self. Think of yourself as independent of the body and as able to leave it without impairing the individuality. You will gradually experience a feeling of blissful rest and calm and content. The attention must, be withdrawn entirely from the physical body and centred entirely upon the higher " I," which is really " you." Think of the vast worlds around us, the millions of suns, each surrounded with its group of planets like our earth, only in many cases much larger. Get an idea of the immensity of space and of time ; consider the extent of Life in all its forms in all these worlds and then realize the position of the earth and of yourself a mere insect upon a speck of dirt. Then rise upward in your thought and realize that, though you be but an atom of the mighty whole, you are still a bit of Life itself, a particle of the Spirit ; that you are immortal, eternal and indestructible ; a necessary part of the Whole, a part which the Whole cannot get along without, a piece needed to fit into the structure of the Whole. Recognize yourself as in touch with all of Life ; feel the Life of the Whole throbbing through you ; the whole ocean of Life rocking you on its bosom. And then awake and return to your physical life and you will find that your body is refreshed, your mind calm and strong, and you will feel an inclination to do that piece of work which you have been putting off for so long. You have profited and been strengthened by your trip into the upper regions of the mind.

A Moment's Rest

A favourite Yogi plan for snatching a moment's rest from the task of the hour—taking rest "on the fly," as one of our young friends recently expressed it—is as follows:

Stand up straight, with head erect and shoulders thrown back, your arms hanging loosely by your sides. Then raise your heels slowly from the ground, gradually throwing your weight upon the balls of the feet, and at the same time raising your arms up by your sides until they stand out from your shoulders like the outstretched wings of an eagle. Take a deep breath as the weight falls upon the balls of the feet and as the arms spread out and you will feel like flying. Then expel the breath slowly and gradually sink back upon the heels and let the arms sink to their first position. Repeat if you like the sensation. The rising and extending of the arms will impart a feeling of buoyancy and freedom that must be experienced to be realized.

CHAPTER XXIV

THE USE OF PHYSICAL EXERCISE

MAN in his original state did not need to be instructed in physical exercise—neither does a child or youth with normal tastes. Man's original state of living gave him an abundance of varied activity out of doors, and with all the best conditions for exercise. He was compelled to seek his food, to prepare it, to raise his crops, to build his houses, to gather up fuel, and to do the thousand and one things which were necessary to live in simple comfort. But as man began to be civilized he also began to delegate certain of his duties to others, and to confine himself to one set of activities, until at the present day many of us do practically no physical work, while others do nothing but hard physical work of a limited scope —both living unnatural lives.

Physical labour without mental activity dwarfs a man's life—and mental labour without some sort of physical activity also dwarfs the man's life. Nature demands the maintaining of the balance—the adoption of the happy medium. The natural, normal life calls for the use of all of man's powers, mental and physical, and the man who is able to so regulate his life that he gets both mental and physical exercise is apt to be the healthiest and happiest.

Children obtain the necessary exercise in their

plays, and the natural instinct of the child causes it to indulge in games and sports. Men, if they are wise, vary their mental labour and sedentary lives with sports and games. The success which has attended the introduction of golf and kindred games of recent years, shows that the old natural instinct of man is not dead.

The Yogis hold that the instinct toward games—the feeling that exercise is needed, is but the same instinct that causes man to labour at congenial occupations—it is the call of nature toward activity—varied activity. The normal, healthy body is a body that is equally well nourished in all of its parts, and no part is properly nourished unless it is used. A part that is unused receives less than the normal amount of nourishment, and in time becomes weakened. Nature has provided man with exercise for every muscle and part of his body, in natural work and play. By natural work, we do not mean the work attendant upon some particular form of bodily labour, for a man following one trade only exercises one set of muscles, and is apt to become "muscle-bound," and is in as much need of exercise as the man who sits at his desk all day, with the exception that the man working at his trade usually has the advantage of more out-of-door life.

We consider the modern plans of "Physical Culture" very poor substitutes for out-of-door work and play. They have no interest attached to them, and the mind is not called into play as it is in the case of work or games. But still anything in the way of exercise is better than nothing. But we protest against that form of Physical Culture which has for its object the enlargement of certain muscles, and the performance of the feats of the "strong men." All this is unnatural. The perfect system of physical culture is that one which tends to produce a uniform development of the entire body—the employment of all the muscles—the nourishment of every part, and which adds as much interest as possible to the exercise, and which keeps its pupils out in the open air.

The Yogis, in their everyday life, do their own work, and get much exercise in this way. They also take long walks through the woods (if they are near woods, and they usually are, for they prefer mountainous country and keep away from the plains and large cities so far as is possible), and over the hills. But they also have a number of forms of mild exercise with which they vary their hours of study and meditation. There is nothing especially novel or new about their exercise, and they bear a very close resemblance to the calisthentic exercises and Delsarte movements in favour in the West. The principal and important point of difference, however, lies in the fact that they use the mind in connection with the bodily movements. Just as the interest in the work, and the game, brings the mind into play, so does the Yogi allow his exercise to call into operation his mind. He takes an interest in the exercises, and by an effort of the will sends an increased flow of prana to the part brought into motion. He thus obtains a multiplied benefit, and a few minutes' exercise do him as much good as would ten times that amount of exercise, if performed in the usual indifferent, uninterested way.

This "knack" of sending the mind to the desired part is easily acquired. All that is necessary is to accept as a fact the statement that it can be done, thus doing away with all sub-conscious resistance, occasioned by the doubting mental attitude; then simply command the mind to send a supply of prana to the part, and to increase the circulation there. The mind does this to a certain extent, involuntarily, the moment that the attention is centred on a part of the body, but the effect is greatly increased by the effort of the will. Now, it is not necessary to contract the brows, clench the fist, or to make a violent physical effort in order to operate the Will in this way. In fact, the simplest way to accomplish the desired result is to *confidently expect* that what you wish will happen. This "confident expectation" acts practically as a strong and positive command of the Will—put it into operation and the thing is accomplished.

For instance, if you wish to send an increased amount of prana to the forearm, and to increase the circulation to that part, thereby increasing the nourishment, simply double the arm, and then gradually extend it, fastening the gaze or attention upon the lower arm, and holding the thought of the desired result. Do this several times, and you will feel that the forearm has been greatly exercised, although you have used no violent motion, and have used no apparatus. Try this plan on several parts of the body, making some muscular motion in order to get the attention there, and you will soon acquire the knack, so that when you go through any ordinary simple exercise you will do this almost automatically.

In short, when you exercise, realize what you are doing and what you are doing it for, and you will get the result. Put life and interest into your exercise, and avoid the listless, mechanical manner of going through the motions, so common in physical culture exercises. Put some " fun " into it, and enjoy it. In this way both mind and body obtain a benefit, and you will leave your exercise with a splendid glow and thrill such as you have not experienced for many a day.

In our next chapter we give a few simple exercises, which if followed will give you all the movements necessary to exercise your entire body, bringing every part into play, strengthening every organ, and making you not only well developed, but straight and erect as an Indian, and as supple and quick of movement as an athlete. These exercises are taken in part from some of the Oriental movements, adapted for Western use, combined with a number of motions which have found favour with the physical trainers of the armies of Europe and America. These army physical directors have studied the Oriental movements, and have adopted such of them as suited their purpose, and have succeeded in forming a series of movements which, while very simple and easily performed in a few minutes, are capable of accomplishing as much for a man or woman as many elaborate courses and systems of physical culture which are sold at high prices. Do not let the simplicity and brevity of this system cause you to undervalue it. It is just the thing you have been looking for, with all the unnecessary features " trimmed off." Try the exercises for a while, before you make up your mind about them. They will practically " make you over " physically, if you will take the time and trouble to put them into faithful practice.

CHAPTER XXV

SOME YOGI PHYSICAL EXERCISES

BEFORE telling you about these exercises, we wish again to impress upon you that exercise without interest fails in its effect. You must manage to take an interest in your exercise, and to throw some mind into it. You must learn to like the work, and to think of what it all means. By following this advice you will obtain multiplied benefit from this work.

STANDING POSITION

Each exercise must be begun by you standing in a natural manner, *i.e.*, with your heels together; head erect; eyes front; shoulders back; chest expanded; abdomen drawn in a little; arms at the sides.

EXERCISE I

(1) Extend the arms straight out in front of you, on the level of the shoulder, with palms of the hands touching each other. (2) Swing back the hands until the arms stand out straight, sideways, from the shoulders, or even a little further back if they will go there easily without forcing; return briskly to Position 1, and repeat several times. The arms should be swung with a rapid movement, and with animation and life. Do not go to sleep over the work, or rather play. This exercise is most useful in developing the chest, muscles of the shoulders,

etc. In swinging the hands backward, it is an improvement if you will rise on your toes during the backward sweep, sinking on your heels as you move the arms forward again. The repeated movements should be rhythmical, backward and forward, like the swinging of a quick pendulum.

Exercise II

(1) Extend the arms straight out from the shoulder, sideways, with opened hands. (2) With the arms so extended, swing the hands around in circles (not too wide), keeping the arms back as far as possible, and not allowing the hands to pass in front of the line of the breast while making the circles. Continue making the circles until say twelve are made. It improves this exercise to inhale a full breath (according to the Yogi practice) and to retain the air until several circles are made. This exercise develops the chest and shoulders, and back. Put life into it, and take an interest in what you are doing.

Exercise III

(1) Extend the arms straight in front of you, letting the little fingers of each hand touch each other, the palms being upward. (2) Then, keeping the little fingers still touching, bring the hands straight up in a curved circular movement, until the tips of the fingers of both hands touch the top of the head back of the forehead, the backs of the fingers touching, the elbows swinging out as the movement is made until (when the fingers touch the head, with thumbs pointing to the rear) they point out straight

sideways. (3) Let the fingers rest on the top of the head a moment, and then with the elbows pressing back (which forces the shoulders back) force the arms backward with an oblique motion until they reach the sides at full length, as in the standing position.

EXERCISE IV

(1) Extend the arms straight out, sideways, from the shoulders. (2) Then, still keeping the upper-arms extended in same position, bend the arms at the elbow and bring the forearm upward with a circular movement, until the tips of the extended fingers lightly touch the tops of the shoulders. (3) Then, keeping the fingers in the last position, force the elbows out to the front until they touch, or nearly so. (A little practice will enable you to touch them together.) (4) Then, keeping the fingers still lightly touching the tops of the shoulders, swing the elbows as far back as you can get them. (A little practice will enable you to get them much further back than at the first attempt.) (5) Swing the elbows to the front position and then back to the rear position, several times.

EXERCISE V

(1) Place the hands on the hips, thumbs to the rear, and elbows pressed back. (2) Bend the body forward, from the hips, as far as you can, keeping the chest protruding and the shoulders pressed back. (3) Raise the body to the original standing position (hands still at hips) and then bend backward. In these movements the knees should not be bent, and

the motions should be made slowly and gently. (4) Then (hands still on hips) bend gently to the right, keeping the heels firmly on the ground, knees unbent, and avoid twisting the body. (5) Resume original position, and then bend the body gently to the left, observing the precautions given in last movement. This exercise is somewhat fatiguing, and you should be careful not to overdo it at the start. Proceed gradually. (6) With hands in same position on the hips, swing the upper part of the body around in a circle, from the waist up, the head describing the largest circle, of course. Do not move the feet or bend the knees.

Exercise VI

(1) Standing erect, raise the arms straight up over the head, hands remaining open with thumbs touching each other when the arms are fully extended upward—palms to the front, of course. (2) Then, without bending the knees, bend the body forward from the waist and endeavour to touch the floor with the extended finger tips—if you are unable to do this at first, do the best you can, and you will soon be able to do it properly—but remember that neither the knees nor the arms must be bent. (3) Rise, and repeat several times.

Exercise VII

(1) Standing erect, with hands on hips, raise yourself on the balls of the feet several times, with sort of a springy motion. Pause a moment after you have raised upon your toes, then let the heels sink to the floor, then repeat, as above suggested.

Keep the knees unbent, and the heels together. This exercise is specially beneficial in developing the calf of the leg, and will make it feel sore the first few times it is tried. If you have an undeveloped calf, here is the exercise for you. (2) With hands still on hips, place your feet about two feet apart, and then lower the body into a "squatting" position, pausing a moment and then resuming original position. Repeat several times, but not too often at first, as it will make the thighs feel a little sore at the beginning. This exercise will give one well developed thighs. This last movement may be improved upon by sinking down with the weight resting upon the ball of the foot, instead of upon the heel.

Exercise VIII

(1) Stand erect, with hands on hips. (2) Keeping the knee straight, swing the right leg out about fifteen inches (keeping the toe turned a little out, and the sole flat), then swing back to the rear until the toe points straight to the ground, *keeping the knee stiff all the time.* (3) Repeat the swinging backward and forward several times. (4) Then do the same with the left leg. (5) With hands still on hips, raise the right leg up, bending the knee, until the upper-leg (thigh) stands straight out from the body (if you can raise it still a little higher, you may do so). (6) Place your foot again on the ground, and go through the same motion with the left leg. (7) Repeat several times, first one leg and then the other, moving slowly at first and gradually increasing your speed until you are executing a slow trot without moving from the one spot.

Exercise IX

(1) Stand erect, with the arms extended straight in front of you, from the shoulders, and of course on a level with the shoulders—the palms must be down, fingers straight out, thumbs folded under, and the thumb side of hands touching each other. (2) Bend the body forward from the hips, stooping forward as far as possible, and at the same time swing the arms forward with a sweeping movement, sending them down, backward and upward at the back, so that when the body has reached the limit of the bending forward movement the arms are extended back and over the body—keep the arms stiff, and do not bend the knees. (3) Resume standing position and repeat several times.

Exercise X

(1) Extend the arms straight, sideways, from the shoulder, and hold them there stiff and rigid with hands open. (2) Close the hands forcibly, with a quick motion, pressing the fingers well into the palm. (3) Open the hands forcibly, and quickly, spreading out the fingers and thumbs as widely as possible, forming a fan-shaped hand. (4) Close and open the hands as above stated, several times, as rapidly as possible. Put life into the exercise. This is a splendid exercise for developing the muscles of the hand, and for acquiring manual dexterity.

Exercise XI

(1) Lie upon your stomach, extending your arms above your head and then bowed upward, and your

legs stretched out full length and raised backward and upward. The correct position may be carried in the mind by imagining a watch-crystal or a saucer resting on the table on its middle, with both ends turning upward. (2) Lower and raise the arms and legs, several times. (3) Then turn over on your back, and lie extended at full length, with arms extended straight out, upward over the head, with back of fingers touching the ground. (4) Then raise up both legs from the waist until they stand straight up in the air, like the mast of a ship, your upper-body and arms remaining in the last position named. Lower the legs and raise them several times. (5) Resume position 3, lying flat upon the back at full length with arms extended straight out upward, over the head, with backs of fingers touching the ground. (6) Then gradually raise body to sitting position, with arms projecting straight out in front of the shoulders. Then go back gradually to the lying-down position, and repeat the rising and lowering several times. (7) Then turn over on the face and stomach again, and assume the following position: Keeping the body rigid from head to foot, raise your body until its weight rests upon your palms (the arms being stretched out straight in front of you) at one end, and upon your toes at the other end. Then gradually bend arms at the elbow, allowing your chest to sink to the floor; then raise up your chest and upper-body by straightening out your arms, the entire weight falling upon the arms, with the toes as a pivot—this last is a difficult motion, and should not be overdone at first.

Exercise to Reduce Large Abdomen

This exercise is for those troubled with a too large abdomen, which trouble is caused by too much fat gathering there. The abdomen may be materially reduced by a reasonable indulgence in this exercise—but always remember "moderation in all things," and do not overdo matters, or be in too much of a hurry. Here is the exercise: (1) Exhale the breath (breathe out all the air in the lungs, without straining yourself too much), and then draw the abdomen in and up as far as you can, then hold for a moment and let it resume its natural position. Repeat a number of times and then take a breath or two, and rest a moment. Repeat several times, moving it in and out. It is surprising how much control one may gain over these stubborn muscles with a little practice. This exercise will not only reduce the fatty layers over the abdomen, but will also greatly strengthen the stomach muscles. (2) Give the abdomen a good (but not rough) kneading and rubbing.

A "Setting-up" Exercise

This exercise is intended to give one a graceful and natural manner of standing and walking, and to cure him of the habit of "slouching," and shambling along. If faithfully practised it will cause you to manifest an erect, graceful carriage. It enables you to so carry yourself that every organ has plenty of "elbow-room," and every part of the frame is properly poised and counter-poised. This, or a similar plan, is followed by the military authorities of many countries, in order to give their young officers the proper carriage, but its good effect in these cases is somewhat marred by other military practices which cause a stiffness which does not come to those who practise this exercise apart from the drill. The exercise is as follows—follow it carefully: (1) Stand erect, with heels together, toes slightly pointed outward. (2) Raise the arms up by the sides (with a circular movement) until the hands meet over the head, thumbs touching each other. (3) Keeping knees stiff; the body rigid; *the elbows unbent* (and shoulders bent well back as the movement is made); bring down the hands, slowly, with a sideway circular motion, until they reach the sides of the legs the little finger and the inner-edge (the "chopping-edge") of the hand alone touching the leg, and the palms of the hands facing straight to the front. The soldier gets the right position by touching the little finger of each hand to the seam of his trousers. (4) Repeat several times, *slowly*, remember. With the hands in the last position, having been placed there by the motion stated, it is very difficult for the shoulders to warp forward. The chest is projected a little; the head is erect; neck is straight; the back straight and hollowed a little (the natural position); and the knees are straight. In short, you have a fine, erect carriage—*now keep it.* It will help you to stand in this position, and then, keeping the little finger along the trouser-leg seam place, walk around the room. A little practice of this kind will work wonders with you, and you will be surprised at the improvement which you have wrought upon yourself. But it takes practice, and perseverance—and so does everything else worth having.

Now this is about all of our little system of exercises. It is simple and unpretentious, but wonderfully effective. It brings every part of the body into play, and if faithfully followed will indeed "make you over" physically. Practise faithfully, and take an interest in the work. Put some mind into it, and remember always what you are doing the work (or play) for. Carry the thought of "STRENGTH AND DEVELOPMENT" with you when you exercise, and you will get much better results. Do not exercise soon after a meal, or immediately before one. Do not overdo things—start with a few repetitions of any exercise at first, and then gradually increase it until you have reached a fair number of repetitions. Better go through the exercises several times a day (if possible) rather than attempt to do too much at one period of exercise.

The above little "Physical Culture" system will do as much for you as will many high priced "courses" of instruction—either personal or by mail. They have stood the test of time, and still are "up-to-date." They are as simple as they are effective. Try them, and be strong.

CHAPTER XXVI

THE YOGI BATH

It should not be necessary to devote a chapter of this book to the importance of bathing. But even in this, the twentieth, century a great mass of the people understand practically nothing about this subject. In the large cities the easy access to the bath-tub has, in a measure, educated the people up to at least a partial use of water on the outer surface of the body, but in the country, and even in many homes in the cities, bathing is not given the place it should occupy in the daily life of the people. And so we think it well to call the attention of our readers to the subject and explain to them why the Yogis set so much store upon a clean body.

In the state of nature man did not need the frequent use of the bath, for, his body being uncovered, the rains beat upon him, and the bushes and trees brushed against his skin, keeping it free from the gathered-up waste matter which the skin is continuously throwing off. And, then, the primitive man, like the animals, always had streams handy, and followed his natural instinct, which impelled him to take a plunge once in a while. But the use of clothing has changed all this, and man to-day, although his skin is still at work throwing off waste matter, is unable to get rid of the waste in the old way, and instead he allows it to pile up on his skin and consequently suffers physical discomfort and disease. A body may be very dirty indeed and still look clean to the naked eye. A peep at the garbage piles on its surface through a strong glass would shock many of you.

Bathing has been practised by all races of men making any pretence of culture and civilization. In fact, it may be said that the use of the bath is a measuring-rod by which the culture of a nation may be determined. The greater the use of the bath, the greater the amount of culture, and the fewer the baths, the less culture. The ancient people carried the use of the bath to a ridiculous extent, departing from the natural methods and running to such extremes as perfumed baths, etc. The Greeks and Romans made the use of the bath a requisite of decent living, and many of the ancient people were far ahead of modern races in this respect. The Japanese people to-day lead the world in the recognition of the importance of the bath and in its faithful practice. The poorest Japanese would rather go without his meal than without his bath. One may go into a crowd in a Japanese city even on a warm day and fail to notice even the slightest unpleasant odour. Would that as much could be said of a crowd in America or Europe ! With many races bathing was, and is to-day, a matter of religious duty, the priests recognizing the importance of bathing, and knowing that it could be best impressed upon the masses in this way, having incorporated it among their religious rites. The Yogis, while not regarding it as a religious rite, nevertheless practise bathing just as if it were.

Let us see just why people should bathe. Very few of us really understand the matter and think it is merely to get rid of the dust and visible dirt which has accumulated upon our skin. But there is more than this to it, important as mere cleanliness is. Let us see just why the skin needs to be cleansed.

We have explained to you, in another chapter, the importance of a normal perspiration and how, if the pores of the skin become clogged or closed, the body is unable to get rid of its waste products. And how does it get rid of them? By the skin, breath and the kidneys. Many persons overwork their kidneys by making them do both their own work and that of the skin as well, for nature will make one organ do double work rather than to leave its work undone. Each pore is the end of a little canal called a sweat-tube, which extends way down into the surface of the body. There are about 3,000 of these little canals to each square inch of our skin. They are continually exuding a moisture called perspiration, or sweat, which moisture is really a fluid secreted from the blood and laden with the impurities and waste matter of the system. You will remember that the body is constantly tearing down tissue and replacing it with new matter, and it must get rid of its waste just as a family must get rid of its waste sweepings and garbage. And the skin is one of the means by which the waste is removed. This waste, if allowed to remain in the system, acts as a breeding-place and food for bacteria, germs, etc., and that is why nature is so anxious to get rid of it. The skin also exudes an oily fluid which is used to keep the skin soft and flexible.

The skin itself is constantly undergoing great changes in its structure, just as is any other part of the body. The outer skin, often called the scarf-skin, is composed of cells, which are short-lived, and are constantly being sloughed off and replaced by younger cells forcing their way up from beneath the old ones. These worn-out and discarded cells form a coating of waste matter on the surface of the skin, if they are not brushed off or washed off. Of course quite a number of them are rubbed off by the clothing, but a considerable quantity remain, and the bath or a wash is needed to get rid of them.

In our chapter on the use of water as an irrigator for the internal man, we told you of the importance of keeping the pores open, and how soon a man would die if his pores were sealed, as shown by experiments and occurrences in the past. And this accumulation of worn-out cells, oil, perspiration, etc., will at least partially seal up the pores unless the body is kept clean. And then, again, this filth on the surface of the skin is an invitation for stray germs and bacteria to take up their abode there and thrive. Are you extending this invitation to your friends, the germs? We are not speaking of dirt obtained from the outside world now—we know that you would not carry that around with you—but have you ever thought of this waste matter from your own system, which is just as much dirt as the other, and sometimes occasions worse results?

Everyone should wash off his body at least once a day. We do not mean that a bath-tub is necessary (although a tub is, of course, a great convenience), but a good wash-off is requisite. Those who have not a bath-tub can get just as good results by taking a towel and a basin and passing the wet towel over the entire body, rinsing the towel after the first rub, and then going over the body the second time.

The most desirable time for a wash-off or a bath is in the early morning, immediately after arising. The evening bath is also a good thing. Never bathe immediately before, or immediately after, a meal. Give the body a good rubbing with a rough cloth, which will act to loosen up the dead skin, and which will also stimulate the circulation. Never take a cold bath when the body is cold. Exercise yourself a little until you warm up some, before taking a cold bath. In taking a plunge bath, always wet the head before getting the body under water—then wet the chest, and then plunge in.

A favourite Yogi practice after taking a cold bath, or a cool one, is to rub the body vigorously with the hands, instead of using a towel, and then getting into dry clothes with the body still covered with moisture. Instead of this making one feel cold, as some might imagine, it produces just the opposite effect, for a feeling of warmth is experienced immediately after the clothing is on, which is increased by a gentle exercise, which the Yogis always take immediately after the bath. This exercise is not violent, and is discontinued as soon as one feels himself in a gentle glow all over the body.

The favourite Yogi bath, or wash-off, is in cool (not *cold*) water. They wash themselves vigorously all over, with the hands, or a cloth, followed by a hand-rubbing, *practising the Yogi deep breathing during the wash and the rubbing.* They take this immediately after arising, and follow it with a mild exercise as we have stated. In very cold weather they do not plunge into the water, but apply it with a cloth, followed by the hand-rubbing. A wonderful reaction follows the application of cool water, applied as we have stated, and the body soon manifests a magnetic glow after the clothing is placed on one after the bath. The result of these Yogi baths if practised for awhile is that the person will become vigorous and "hardy," their flesh becoming strong, firm and compact, and a "cold" becoming almost unknown to them. The person practising it becomes like a strong, hardy tree, able to face all kinds of weather and seasons.

Right here, let us caution our readers against adopting a too cold bath at the start. Don't do this, particularly if you are of impaired vitality. Try water at a pleasant temperature at first, and then work down toward a little cooler, gradually. You will soon strike a degree of temperature that is most pleasing to you—stick to that. But do not punish yourselves. This morning cool wash-down should be a thing of pleasure to you, not a punishment or a penance. When you have once caught the "knack" of it, you would never think of giving it up. It makes you feel good all day long. You feel a little cool as the wet cloth is applied to the body, but this is followed in a moment or so by a most delightful reaction and a feeling of warmth. In case you take a cool bath in the tub, instead of a wash-down, do not stay in the tub more than one minute, and use your hands vigorously the whole time that you are in the water.

If you take these morning washes, you will not need many warm baths, although an occasional "soaking" will do you good, and you will feel better for it. Give yourself a good rubbing down, and put on the clothing over a dry skin (in the case of a *warm* bath).

Persons doing much walking, or standing, will find that a foot bath at night just before retiring will prove most restful, and conducive to a good night's sleep.

Now don't forget this chapter as soon as you have read it, but try the plan it advocates, and see how much better you will feel. After trying it for awhile, you will not think of giving it up.

The Yogi Morning Wash-down

The following may give you some ideas regarding the way to get the best results from the morning wash-down. It is very invigorating and strengthening, and will make one feel the beneficial effect all the day.

It begins with a little exercise which causes the blood to circulate and the Prana to be distributed all over the body, after the night's rest, and renders the body in the best condition in which to take the cool wash-down or bath.

Preliminary Exercise. (1) Stand erect in a military attitude, head up, eyes front, shoulders back, hands at sides. (2) Raise the body slowly on toes, inhaling a deep breath, steadily and slowly. (3) Retain the breath for a few seconds, maintaining the same position. (4) Sink slowly to the first position, at the same time exhaling the breath through the nostrils, slowly. (5) Practise Cleansing Breath. (6) Repeat several times, varying by using right leg alone, then left leg alone.

Then take the bath or wash-down, as described on the preceding pages. If you prefer the wash-down, fill the basin with cool water (not too cool, but just a pleasant stimulating temperature which will bring on the reaction). Take a rough cloth or towel and soak it in the water, and then wring about half the water out of it. Beginning with the chest and shoulders, then the back, then the abdomen, then the thighs and then the lower legs and feet, rub the body all over vigorously. Wring the water out of the towel several times in going over the body, in order that the entire body shall receive fresh cool water upon it. Pause a second or so several times during the wash-down, and take a couple of long deep breaths. Do not be in too much of a rush, but go about it calmly. At first few times the cool water may cause you to shrink a little, but you will soon get used to it, and will learn to like it. Do not make the mistake of commencing with too cool water, but rather work down the temperature by degrees. If you prefer the tub to the wash-down, half fill the tub with water of the proper temperature, and kneel in it while you do the rubbing, then plunge the whole body under the water for a moment, and then get out at once.

Following either the wash-down or the tubbing, one should rub the hands vigorously over the body several times. There is something in the human hands which cannot be duplicated by a cloth or towel. Try it for yourself. Leave a little moisture on the surface of the skin, and then get into your underclothes at once, and you will be surprised at the peculiar glow which will come over you. Instead of the water making you feel chilly you will experience a peculiar feeling of warmth on all parts of the body covered by the clothing, under which a little moisture has been left on the skin. In case of either wash-down or tubbing, follow the wash or bath with the following exercise, after the underclothing has been put on:

Concluding Exercise. (1) Stand erect; stretch out arms straight in front of you, on the level of the shoulders, with fists clenched and touching each other; swing back the fists until the arms stand out straight, sideways, from the shoulders (or still a little farther back if they will go there easily without forcing)—this stretches the upper part of the chest; repeat several times and then rest a moment. (2) Resume the closing position of 1, the arms straight out, sideways, from the shoulders; the arms still extending from the sides, on a level with the shoulders, swing the fists around in circles, from the front to the back—then reverse, and swing from the back to the front—then vary it by rotating them alternately, like the arms of a windmill; repeat several times. (3) Stand erect, raise the hands over the head; hands open, and thumbs touching; then without bending the knees try to touch the floor with the tips of the fingers—if you are unable to do this, do the best you can; return to first position. (4) Raise yourself on the balls of your feet, or your toe-joints, several times, with sort of a springy motion. (5) Standing, place your feet about two feet apart, then sink slowly to a squatting position, for a moment, then resume original position. Repeat several times. (6) Repeat No. 1, several times. (7) Finish with the Cleansing Breath.

This exercise is not nearly as complicated as it appears at first reading. It is really a combination of five exercises, all of which are very simple and easily performed. Study and practise each section of the exercise, before you take the bath, and master each part thoroughly. Then it will run like clock-work, and will take but a few moments to perform it. It is very invigorating, calling into play the entire body, and will make you feel like a new man, or woman, if you take it just after the bath or wash-down.

The wash-down of the upper part of the body in the morning, gives a strength and vitality through the day, while a wash-down of the body from the waist down (including the feet) at night, rests one for the night's slumber, and is very refreshing.

CHAPTER XXVII

THE SOLAR ENERGY

OUR students are, of course, more or less familiar with the fundamental scientific principles of astronomy. That is to say, they are aware that even in that infinitesimally small portion of the Universe of which we have any knowledge through the sense of sight, even when aided by the most powerful telescopes, there are millions of fixed stars—all of which are suns, equal in size to, and in some cases many times larger than the sun governing our particular planetary system. Each sun is a centre of energy for its planetary system. Our sun is the greater radiator of energy for our planetary system, which is composed of several planets known to science, and several still unknown to astronomers—our own planet, the Earth, being but one of a large family.

Our sun, like the other suns, is continually throwing off energy into space, which energy vitalizes its surrounding planets and makes life possible on them. Without the rays of the sun, life would be impossible on the earth—even the most simple forms of life known to us. We are all dependent upon the sun for vitality—vital force. This vital force or energy is of course that which the Yogis know as Prana. Prana is of course everywhere, yet certain centres are constantly being used to absorb and again send this energy—to keep up a perpetual current as it were. Electricity is everything, but still dynamos and like centres are necessary to gather it up and send it out in concentrated form. A constant current of Prana is maintained between the sun and its several planets.

It is generally taken for granted (and modern science does not dispute it) that the sun is a mass of seething fire—a sort of fiery furnace, and that the light and heat which we receive are the emanations from this great furnace. But the Yogi philosophers have always held differently. They teach that although the constitution of the sun, or rather the conditions prevailing there, are so different from those prevailing here that the human mind would have much difficulty in forming an intelligent conception of them, still it is not literally a mass of matter in combustion, just as a blazing ball of burning coal would be—nor is it as a ball of molten iron. Neither of these conceptions is accepted by the Yogi teachers. They hold, on the contrary, that the sun is composed largely of certain substances very similar to the newly discovered substance known as "radium." They do not say that the sun is composed of radium, but have held for many centuries that it is composed of numerous substances, or forms of matter, having properties similar to those observed to exist in that substance which the Western world is just now thinking so much about, and which its discoverers have termed radium. We are not attempting to describe or explain radium, but are merely stating that it seems to possess certain qualities and properties which the Yogis teach are possessed in varying degrees by the several substances forming the "sun-matter." It is very probable that some of the other sun-substances may yet be found on this planet—resembling radium and yet having points of difference.

This sun-substance is not in a molten state, or in a state of combustion as we generally use the word. But it is constantly drawing to itself a current of Prana from the planets, passing it through some wonderful process of Nature and sending a return current to the planets. As our students know, the air is the principal source from which we extract Prana, but the air itself receives it from the sun. We have told how the food we eat is filled with Prana, which we extract and use—but the plants receive their Prana from the sun. The sun is the great storehouse of Prana for this solar system, and is a mighty dynamo constantly sending forth its vibrations to the limits of its system, vitalizing everywhere and making possible life—physical life, we mean, of course.

This book is not the place in which to attempt to describe the wonderful facts regarding the sun's work, which are known to the best Yogi teachers, and we touch upon the subject merely that our students will know the sun for what it is, and realize what it means to all living creatures. The object of this chapter is to bring to your minds the fact that the sun's rays are filled with vibrations of energy and life, which we are using every moment of our lives, but which we are most likely not using to the degree possible to us. Modern and civilized people seem afraid of the sun—they darken their rooms, cover themselves all over with heavy clothes in order to keep out its rays—run away from it, in fact. Now, remember right here that when we speak of the sun's rays we are not speaking of *heat*. Heat is produced by the action of the sun's rays coming in contact with the earth's atmosphere—outside of the earth's atmosphere (in the inter-planetary regions) intense cold prevails, because there is no resistance offered the sun's rays. So when we tell you to take advantage of the sun's rays, we do not mean to sit out in the heat of the mid-summer sun.

You must stop this practice of running away from the sunlight. You must admit the sun to your rooms. Do not be so afraid of your rugs or carpets. Do *not* keep your best rooms closed all the time. You do not wish your rooms to be like a cellar into which the sun never shines. Open your windows in the early morning, and let the rays of the sun, either direct or reflected, beat into the room, and you will find an atmosphere of health, strength and vitality gradually pervading your home, replacing the old atmosphere of disease, weakness and lack of life.

Get out into the sun once in awhile—don't shun the sunny side of the street, except when the weather is very warm indeed, or about noon-time. Take sun-baths occasionally. Get up a few minutes earlier, and stand, sit or lie down in the sun, and let it freshen up your whole body. If you are so situated that you may do so, take off your clothing and let the sun's rays reach your body without the interference of clothing. If you have never tried this, you will scarcely believe how much virtue there is in a sun-bath, and how strong you will feel after it. Do not dismiss this subject without a thought. Experiment a little with the sun's rays, and get some of the benefit of the direct vibrations on your body. If you have any special weakness of the body, you will find that you will obtain relief by letting the rays of the sun reach the affected part, or the surface of the body right over the affected part.

The early morning rays of the sun are by far the most beneficial, and those who rise early and get the benefit of these fresh rays are to be congratulated. After the sun has risen about five hours, the vital effects of the rays lessen, and then gradually decrease as the day nears its close. You will notice that flower-beds which receive the early morning sunshine, thrive much better than those who get only the afternoon rays. All lovers of flowers understand this, and realize that sunshine is as necessary to healthy plant life, as is water, air and good soil. Study the plants a little—get back to nature, and read your lesson there. The sun and air are wonderful tonics—why do you not partake of them more freely?

In other parts of this book, we have spoken of the power of the mind to attract to the system an additional share of Prana from the air, food, water, etc. And this is true of the Prana or vital force in the sun's rays—you may increase the benefit by the proper mental attitude. Walk out in the morning sun—lift up your head, throw back your shoulders, take a few good breaths of the air which is being charged with Prana from the sun's rays. Let the sun shine on you. And then, form the mental image suggested by the words, while you repeat the following (or similar) mantram: "I am bathed in Nature's beautiful sunlight—I am drawing from it life, health, strength and vitality. It is making me strong and full of energy. I feel the influx of Prana —I feel it coursing all through my system, from my head to my feet, invigorating my entire body. I love the sunlight, and get all its benefits."

Practise this whenever you get an opportunity, and then you will gradually begin to realize what a good thing you have been missing all these years while you have been running away from the sun. Do not unduly expose yourself to the mid-summer sun, on hot days, particularly about noon. But, winter and summer, the early morning rays will not hurt you. Learn to love the sunlight and all that it stands for.

CHAPTER XXVIII

FRESH AIR

Now, do not pass by this chapter because it treats of a very common subject. If you feel inclined to so pass it by—then you are the very person for whom it is intended, and by whom it is most needed. Those who have looked into the matter and have learned something of the benefit and necessity of fresh air, will not pass this chapter by, even though they may know all that it contains—they are glad to read the good news again. And, if you don't like the subject, and feel inclined to skip it, then you surely need it. In other chapters of this book we have spoken of the importance of breathing—both in its esoteric as well as its exoteric phase. This chapter is not intended to take up the subject of breathing again, but will merely give a little preachment upon the necessity of fresh air and plenty of it—a preachment much needed by the people of the West, where hermetically closed sleeping rooms and air-tight houses are so much in vogue. We have told you of the importance of correct breathing, but the lesson will do you but little good unless you have good fresh air to breathe.

This thing of people shutting themselves up in tightly closed rooms, lacking proper ventilation, is the most stupid idea that one can conceive of. How people can do it after acquainting themselves with the facts regarding the action and functions of the lungs, is more than the thinking man can answer. Let us take a plain, common-sense, brief look at this subject.

You will remember that the lungs are constantly throwing off the waste matter of the system—the breath is being used as a scavenger of the body, carrying off the waste products, broken-down and refuse matter from all parts of the system. The matter thrown off by the lungs is almost as foul as that thrown off by the skin, the kidneys and even the bowels—in fact, if the supply of water given the system is not sufficient, nature makes the lungs do much of the work of the kidneys, in getting rid of the foul, poisonous waste products of the body. And if the bowels are not carrying off the normal amount of waste matter, much of the contents of the colon gradually works through the system, seeking an outlet, and is taken up by the lungs and thrown off in the exhaled breath. Just think of it —if you shut yourself up in a tightly closed room, you are pouring out into the atmosphere of that room over eight gallons an hour of carbonic acid gas, and other foul and poisonous gases. In eight hours you throw off sixty-four gallons. If there are two sleeping in the room, multiply the gallons by two. As the air becomes contaminated, you breathe this poisonous matter over and over again into your system, the quality of the air becoming worse with each exhaled breath. No wonder that anyone coming into your room in the morning notices the stench pervading it, if you have kept the windows lowered. No wonder you feel cross, stupid, quarrelsome, and generally " grouchy " after a night in this kind of a pest house.

Did you ever think just why you sleep at all? It is to give nature a chance to repair the waste that has been going on during the day. You cease using up her energies in work, and give her a chance to repair and build up your system so that you will be all right on the morrow. And in order to do this work right, she requires at least normal conditions. She expects to be supplied with air containing the proper proportion of oxygen—air that has been exposed to the sunlight of the preceding day and which has thereby been freshly charged with Prana. Instead of this you give her nothing but a limited amount of air, half-poisoned with the refuse of your body. No wonder she gives you nothing but a patch-work job sometimes.

Any room that smells of that peculiar fetid odour that you have all noticed in a poorly ventilated bedroom, is no place for you to sleep in until it has been ventilated and kept supplied with fresh air. The air in a bedroom should be as nearly as possible kept as pure as the outside air. Don't be afraid of catching cold. Remember that the most approved modern method of treating consumption calls for the patient to be kept in the fresh air, at night, no matter how cold it is. Put on plenty of bed covering, and you will not mind the cold after you get a little used to it Get back to nature! Fresh air does not mean sleeping in a draught, remember.

And what is true of sleeping rooms is also true of living rooms, offices, etc. Of course, in winter one may not allow too much of the outside air to get into the house, as that would bring down the temperature too low, but still there is a happy compromise which may be made even in cold climates. Open the windows once in awhile and give the air a chance to circulate in and out. In the evening, do not forget that the lamps and gaslights are using up a goodly supply of oxygen also—so freshen things up a little, once in awhile. Read up something on ventilation, and your health will be better. But even if you do not care to go that deep into the matter, think a little bit of what we have said, and your common sense will do the rest.

Get out awhile every day and let the fresh air blow upon you. It is full of life and health giving properties. You all know this, and have known it all your lives. But, nevertheless, you stick indoors in a manner which is entirely foreign to nature's plans. No wonder you do not feel well. One cannot violate nature's rules with impunity. Do not be afraid of the air. Nature intended you to use it—it is adapted to your nature and requirements. So don't be afraid of it—learn to love it. Say to yourself while walking out and enjoying the fresh air: "I am a child of Nature—she gives me this pure, good air to use, in order that I may grow strong and well, and keep so. I am breathing in health and strength and energy. I am enjoying the sensation of the air blowing upon me, and I feel its beneficial effects. I am Nature's child, and I enjoy her gifts." Learn to *enjoy* the air, and you will be blessed.

CHAPTER XXIX

NATURE'S SWEET RESTORER—SLEEP

Of all of nature's functions that should be understood by people, sleep seems the one which should be so simple that no instruction or advice should be needed. The child needs no elaborate treatise upon the value and necessity of sleep—it just *sleeps*, that's all. And the adult would do the same if he lived closer to nature's ways. But he has surrounded himself with such artificial environments that it is almost impossible for him to live naturally. But he may go a considerable distance on the return journey to nature, notwithstanding his unfavourable environments.

Of all the foolish practices that man has picked up on his travels away from nature, his habits of sleeping and rising are among the worst. He wastes in excitement and social pleasures the hours which nature has given him for his best sleep, and he sleeps over the hours in which nature has given him the greatest chance to absorb vitality and strength. The best sleep is that taken between the hours of sunset and midnight, and the best hours for out-of-door work and the absorbing of vitality are the first few hours after the sun rises. So we waste at both ends, and then wonder why we break down in middle age or before.

During sleep nature does a great part of her repair

work and it is highly important that she be given this opportunity. We will not attempt to lay down any rules about sleeping, as different people have different needs, and this chapter is merely given as a slight suggestion. Generally speaking, however, about eight hours is the normal demand of nature for sleep.

Always sleep in a well ventilated room, for reasons given in our chapter on fresh air. Place upon yourself enough bed-clothing to keep you comfortable, but do not bury yourself under the mass of heavy bed-clothing that is common in so many families—this is largely a matter of habit, and you will be surprised at how much less bed-clothing you can get along with than you have been using. Never sleep in any garments that you have worn during the day—this practice is neither healthy nor cleanly. Do not pile up too many pillows under your head—one small one is enough. Relax every muscle in the body, and take the tension off of every nerve, and learn to " loaf " in bed, and to cultivate " that lazy feeling " when you get under the covers. Train yourself not to think of the affairs of the day after you retire—make this an invariable rule and you will soon learn to sleep like the healthy child. Watch a child sleep, and what it does after going to bed, and endeavour to follow its plan as nearly as possible. Be a child when you go to bed, and endeavour to live over again the sensations of childhood, and you will sleep like the child—this one piece of advice is worthy of being printed alone in a handsomely bound book, for if followed we would have a race of greatly improved people.

If one has acquired an idea of the real nature of man, and his place in the universe, he will be more likely to drop into this childlike rest than will the average man or woman. He feels so perfectly at home in the universe, and has that calm confidence and trust in the overruling power, that he, like the child, relaxes his body and takes the tension off his mind, and gradually drops off into a peaceful sleep.

We will not give here any special directions regarding the bringing on of sleep to people who have suffered with sleeplessness. We believe that if they will follow the plans for rational and natural living given in this book, they will sleep naturally, without any special advice. But it may be as well to give one or two bits of advice along this line, for the use of those "on the way." Bathing the legs and feet in cool water, just before retiring, produces sleepiness. Concentrating the mind on the feet, has been a help to many, as it directs the circulation to the lower part of the body, and relieves the brain. But above all, do not *try* to go to sleep—this is the worst thing in the world for one who really wishes to sleep, for it generally acts the other way. The better plan, if you think of it at all, is to assume the mental attitude that you do not care whether or not you sleep right off—that you are perfectly relaxed—are enjoying a good "loaf," and are perfectly satisfied with things as they are. Imagine yourself a tired child, resting in a half-drowsy way, not fully asleep nor fully awake, and endeavour to act out this suggestion. Do not bother about later in the night, and whether or not you will sleep then—just live in that particular moment, and enjoy your "loaf."

The exercises given in the chapter on Relaxation will get you into the habit of relaxing at will, and those who have been troubled with sleeplessness will find that they may acquire entirely new habits

Now, we know that we cannot expect all of our students to go to bed like the child, and awaken early like the child, or the farmer. We wish that this were possible, but we realize just what modern life, particularly in the large cities, requires of one. So all that we can ask our students to do is to try to live as closely to nature in this respect as possible. Avoid, so far as you can, late hours and excitement at night, and whenever you get a chance, retire early and rise early. We realize, of course, that all this will interfere with what you have been taught to regard as " pleasure," but we ask that in the midst of this so-called " pleasure " you take a little rest once in awhile. Sooner or later the race will return to more simple manners of living, and late hour dissipation will be regarded as we now regard the use of narcotics, drunkenness, etc. But in the meantime, all that we can say is, "Do the best you can for yourself."

If you are able to get a little time off in the middle of the day, or other times, you will find that a half-hour's relaxation, or even a little " snooze," will do wonders toward refreshing you and enabling you to do better work when you arise. Many of our most successful business and professional men have learned this secret, and many a time when they are reported as being " very busy for a half-hour " they are really lying on their couches, relaxing, breathing deeply, and giving nature a chance to recuperate.

By alternating a little rest with one's work, he will be able to do twice as good work as if he had worked without a break or rest. Think over these things a little, you people of the Western world, and you may be even more "strenuous" by varying your strenuosity by occasional relaxation and rest. A little "letting-go" helps one to take a fresh grip and to hold on all the harder.

CHAPTER XXX

REGENERATION

In this chapter we can but briefly direct your attention to a subject of vital importance to the race, but which the race generally is not ready to seriously consider. Owing to the present state of public opinion upon this subject it is impossible to write as plainly as one would like, or as is really necessary, and all writings upon the subject in question are apt to be considered as "impure," although the only object of the writer may be to counteract the impurity and improper practices indulged by the public. However, some brave writers have managed to give the public a very fair acquaintance with the subject of regeneration, so that the majority of our readers will readily understand what we mean.

We will not take up the important subject of the use of regeneration as applied to the relation of the two sexes, as that subject is so important as to require a volume by itself, and then, besides, this work is scarcely the one in which this subject should be discussed in detail. We will, however, say a few words on the subject. The Yogis regard as wholly unnatural the excesses entered into by the majority of men, and into which they compel their partners in matrimony to join. They believe that the sex-principle is too sacred to be so abused, and feel that man often descends below the level of the brute in his sex relations. With but one or two exceptions the lower animals have sexual relations only for the purpose of perpetuating their kind, and sexual excesses, drains and waste such as man indulges in are almost entirely unknown to the lower animal.

As man has advanced in the scale of life, however, he has brought to light new functions of sex, and there is an interchange of certain higher principles between the sexes, which does not occur to the brutes or to the more material forms of human life—this is reserved for the man and woman of developed mentality and spirituality. Proper relations between husband and wife tend to elevate, strengthen, and ennoble, instead of degrading, weakening, and defiling the participants, as is the case when the said relation is based upon mere sensuality. This is the reason that there is so much marital inharmony and discord when one of the partners rises to a higher plane of thought, and finds that his or her partner is unable to follow. Thereafter their mutual relations are upon different planes, and they fail to find in each other that which they might wish for. This is all we wish to say upon this particular part of the subject here. There are a number of good books upon the subject, that our students may find by inquiring at the centres for advanced thought literature in the different cities and towns. We will confine ourselves in the remainder of this short chapter to the discussion of the subject of the importance of preserving sexual strength and health.

While leading a life in which the actual relations of the sexes do not play an important part, the Yogis recognize and appreciate the importance of healthy reproductive organism, and their effect upon the general health of the individual. With these organs in a weakened condition the entire physical system feels the reflex action and suffers sympathetically. The Complete Breath (described elsewhere in this book) produces a rhythm which is nature's own plan for keeping this important part of the system in normal condition, and, from the first, it will be noticed that the reproductive functions are strengthened and vitalized, thus, by sympathetic reflex action, giving tone to the whole system. By this we do not mean that the animal passions will be aroused—far from it. The Yogis are advocates of continence and chastity, and purity *in* the marriage relation as well as out of it. They have learned to control the animal passions, and to hold them subject to the control of the higher principles of the mind and will. But sexual control does not mean sexual weakness, and the Yogi teachings are that the man or woman whose reproductive organism is normal and healthy will have a stronger will with which to control himself or herself. The Yogi believes that much of the perversion of this wonderful part of the system comes from a lack of normal health and results from a morbid rather than from a normal condition of the reproductive system.

The Yogis also know that the sex-energy may be conserved and used for the development of the body and mind of the individual, instead of being dissipated in unnatural excesses as is the wont of so many uninformed people.

We give in the following pages one of the favourite Yogi exercises for producing this result. Whether or not the student wishes to follow the Yogi theories of clean living, he will find that the Complete Breath will do more to restore health to this part of the system than anything else ever tried. Remember, now, we mean normal health, not undue development. The sensualist will find that normal means a lessening of desire rather than an increase; the weakened man or woman will find that normal means a toning up and relief from the weakness which has heretofore depressed him or her. We do not wish to be misunderstood on this subject. The Yogi's ideal is a body strong in all its parts, and under the control of a masterful and developed will, animated by high ideals.

The Yogis possess great knowledge regarding the use and abuse of the reproductive principle in both sexes. Some hints of this esoteric teaching have filtered out, and have been used by Western writers on the subject, and much good thereby accomplished. In this book we cannot go into a discussion of the underlying theory, but will call your attention to a method whereby the student may be enabled to transmute the reproductive energy into vitality for the whole system instead of wasting it and dissipating it in lustful indulgences. The reproductive energy is creative energy, and may be taken up by the system and transmuted into strength and vitality, thus serving the purpose of regeneration instead of generation. If the young men of the Western world understood these underlying principles, they would be saved much misery and unhappiness in after years, and would be stronger mentally, morally and physically.

This transmutation of the reproductive energy gives great vitality to those practising it. It fills them with great vital force, which will radiate from them and cause them to be known as "magnetic" personalities. The energy thus transmuted may be turned into new channels and used to great advantage. Nature has condensed one of its most powerful manifestations of prana into reproductive energy, as its purpose is to create. The greatest amount of vital force is concentrated into the smallest space. The reproductive organism is the most powerful storage battery in animal life, and its force may be drawn upward and used, as well as expended in the ordinary functions of reproduction, or wasted in riotous lust.

The Yogi exercise for transmuting reproductive energy is simple. It is coupled with rhythmic breathing and is easily performed. It may be practised at any time, but is strongly recommended when one feels the instinct most strongly, at which time the reproductive energy is manifesting, and may be easily transmuted for regenerative purposes. We give it in the next paragraph. The men or women doing mental creative work, or bodily creative work, will be able to use this creative energy in their vocations, by following the exercise, drawing up the energy with each inhalation and sending it forth with the exhalation. The student will understand, of course, that it is not the actual reproductive fluids that are drawn up and used, but the etheric pranic energy which animates the latter—the soul of the reproductive organism, as it were.

Regenerative Exercise

Keep the mind fixed on the idea of Energy and away from ordinary sexual thoughts or imaginings. If these thoughts come into the mind do not feel discouraged, but regard them as manifestations of a force which you intend to use for the purpose of strengthening your body and mind. Lie passively, or sit erect, and fix your mind upon the idea of drawing the reproductive energy upward to the Solar Plexus, where it will be transmuted and stored away as a reserve force of vital energy. Then breathe rhythmically, forming the mental image of drawing up the reproductive energy with each inhalation. With each inhalation make a command of the Will that the energy be drawn upward from the reproductive organism to the Solar Plexus. If the rhythm is fairly established and the mental image is clear, you will be conscious of the upward passage of the energy, and will feel its stimulating effect. If you desire an increase in mental force, you may draw it up to the brain instead of to the Solar Plexus, by giving the mental command and holding the mental image of the transmission to the brain. In this last form of the exercise, only such portions of the energy as may be needed in the mental work being done will pass into the brain, the balance remaining stored up in the Solar Plexus. It is usual to allow the head to bend forward easily and naturally during the transmuting exercise.

This subject of Regeneration opens up a wide field for investigation, research and study, and some day we may find it advisable to issue a little manual upon the subject, for private circulation among the few who are ready for it, and who seek the knowledge from the purest motives, rather than from a desire to find something which will appeal to their lascivious imaginations and inclinations.

CHAPTER XXXI

THE MENTAL ATTITUDE

THOSE who have familiarized themselves with the Yogi teachings regarding the Instinctive Mind and its control of the physical body—and also of the effect of the Will upon the Instinctive Mind—will readily see that the mental attitude of the person will have much to do with his or her health. Bright, cheerful and happy mental attitudes reflect themselves in the shape of normal functioning of the physical body, while depressed mental states, gloom, worry, fear, hate, jealousy, and anger all react upon the body and produce physical inharmony, and eventually disease.

We are all familiar with the fact that good news and cheerful surroundings promote a normal appetite, while bad news, depressing surroundings, etc., will cause the loss of the appetite. The mention of some favourite dish will make the mouth water, and the recollection of some unpleasant experience or sight may produce nausea.

Our mental attitudes are mirrored in our Instinctive Mind, and as that principle of mind has direct control of the physical body, it may readily be understood just how the mental state takes form in the physical action of functioning.

Depressing thought affects the circulation, which in turn affects every part of the body, by depriving it of its proper nourishment. Inharmonious thought destroys the appetite, and the consequence is that the body does not receive the proper nourishment, and the blood becomes impoverished. On the other hand, cheerful, optimistic thought promotes the digestion, increases the appetite, helps the circulation, and, in fact, acts as a general tonic upon the system.

Many persons suppose that this idea of the affect of the mind upon the body is but the idle theory of occultists, and persons interested along the line of mental therapeutics, but one has but to go to the records of scientific investigators to realize that this theory is based upon well established facts. Experiments have been tried, many times, tending to prove that the body is most receptive to the mental attitude or belief, and persons have been made sick, and others cured by simple auto-suggestion or the suggestion of others, which in effect are but strong mental attitudes.

The saliva is rendered a poison under the influence of anger; mother's milk becomes poisonous to the babe if the mother manifests excessive anger or fear. The gastric juice ceases to flow freely if the person becomes depressed or fearful. A thousand instances of this kind could be given.

Do you doubt the fact that disease may be primarily caused by negative thinking? Then listen to the testimony of a few authorities of the Western world.

"Any severe anger or grief is almost certain to be succeeded by fever in certain parts of Africa."—*Sir Samuel Baker, in the "British and Foreign Medico Chirurgical Review."*

"Diabetes from sudden mental shock is a true, pure type of a physical malady of mental origin."—*Sir B. W. Richardson, in "Discourses."*

"In many cases, I have seen reasons for believing that cancer had its origin in prolonged anxiety."—*Sir George Paget, in "Lectures."*

"I have been surprised how often patients with primary cancer of the liver lay the cause of this ill health to protracted grief or anxiety. The cases have been far too numerous to be accounted for as mere coincidences."—*Murchison.*

"The vast majority of cases of cancer, especially of breast or uterine cancer, are probably due to mental anxiety."—*Dr. Snow, in "The Lancet."*

Dr. Wilks reports cases of jaundice resulting from mental conditions. Dr. Churton, in the "British Medical Journal," reports a case of jaundice arising from anxiety. Dr. Makenzie reports several cases of pernicious anaemia caused by mental shock. Hunter reports "an exciting cause of angina pectoris has long been known to be emotional excitement."

"Eruptions on the skin will follow excessive mental strain. In all these, and in cancer, epilepsy, and mania from mental causes, there is a predisposition. It is remarkable how little the question of physical disease from mental influences has been studied."—*Richardson.*

"My experiments show that irascible, malevolent and depressing emotions generate in the system injurious compounds, some of which are extremely poisonous; also that agreeable, happy emotions generate chemical compounds of nutritious value, which stimulate the cells to manufacture energy."—*Elmer Gates.*

Dr. Hack Tuke, in his well known work on mental diseases, etc., written long before the "Mind-cure" interest was manifested in the Western world, gives numerous cases of diseases produced by fear, among them being insanity, idiocy, paralysis, jaundice, premature grayness and baldness, decay of the teeth, uterine troubles, erysipelas, eczema and impetigo.

During times when contagious diseases are prevalent in communities, it is a well attested fact that fear causes a great number of the cases, and also causes many deaths in cases in which the attack is but light. This is readily understood when we consider the fact that contagious diseases are more apt to attack the person manifesting impaired vitality, and the further fact that fear and kindred emotions impair the vitality.

There have been a number of good books written upon this matter, so there is no occasion for us to dwell at length upon this part of the general subject. But before leaving it, we must impress upon our students the truth of the oft repeated statement as "Thought takes form in action," and that mental conditions are reproduced in physical manifestations.

The Yogi Philosophy, in its entirety, tends to produce a mental attitude of calmness, peace, strength and absolute fearlessness among its students, which, of course, is reflected in their physical condition. To such persons mental calmness and fearlessness comes as a matter of course, and no special effort is necessary to produce it. But to those who have not as yet acquired this mental calm, a great improvement may be obtained by the carrying of the thought of the proper mental attitude, and the repetition of mantrams calculated to produce the mental image. We suggest the frequent repetition of the words "BRIGHT, CHEERFUL AND HAPPY," and the frequent contemplation of the meaning of the words. Endeavour to manifest these words into physical action, and you will be greatly benefited both mentally and physically, and will also be preparing your mind to receive high spiritual truths.

CHAPTER XXXII

LED BY THE SPIRIT

WHILE this book is intended to treat solely upon the care of the physical body, leaving the higher branches of the Yogi Philosophy to be dealt with in other writings, still the leading principle of the Yogi teachings is so bound up with the minor branches of the subject, and is so largely taken into account by the Yogis in the simplest acts of their lives, that in justice to the teachings as well as to our students, we cannot leave the subject without at least saying a few words about this underlying principle.

The Yogi Philosophy, as our students doubtless know, holds that man is slowly growing and unfolding, from the lower forms and manifestations to higher, and still higher expressions of the Spirit. Spirit is in each man, although often so obscured by the confining sheaths of his lower nature that it is scarcely discernible. It is also in the lower forms of life, working up and ever seeking for higher forms of expression. The material sheaths of this progressing life—the bodies of mineral, plant, lower animal and man—are but instruments to be used for the best development of the higher principles. But, although the use of the material body is but temporary, and the body itself nothing more than a suit of clothes to be put on, worn, and then discarded, yet it is always the intent of Spirit to provide and maintain as perfect an instrument as possible. It provides the best body possible, and gives the impulses toward right living, but if from causes not to be mentioned here, an imperfect body is provided for the soul, still the higher principles strive to adapt and accommodate themselves to it, and make the best of it.

This instinct of self-preservation—this urge behind all of life—is a manifestation of the Spirit. It works through the most rudimentary forms of the Instinctive Mind up through many stages until it reaches the highest manifestations of that mental principle. It also manifests through the Intellect, in the direction of causing the man to use his reasoning powers for the purpose of maintaining his physical soundness and life. But, alas! the Intellect does not keep to its own work, for as soon as it begins to be conscious of itself it begins to meddle with the duties of the Instinctive Mind, and overriding the instinct of the latter, it forces all sorts of unnatural modes of living upon the body, and seems to try to get as far away from nature as possible. It is like a boy freed from the parental restraint, who goes as far contrary to the parents' example and advice as possible—just to show that he is independent. But the boy learns his folly, and retraces his steps—and so will the Intellect.

Man is beginning to see now, that there is something within him that attends to the wants of his body, and which knows its own business much better than he does. For man with all his Intellect is unable to duplicate the feats of the Instinctive Mind working through the body of the plant, animal or himself. And he learns to trust this mental principle as a friend, and to let it work out its own duties. In the present modes of life which man has seen fit to adopt, in his evolution, but from which he will return to first principles sooner or later, it is impossible to live a wholly natural life, and physical existence must be more or less abnormal as a consequence. But nature's instinct of self-preservation and accommodation is great, and it manages to get along very well with a considerable of a handicap, and does its work much better than one would expect considering the absurd and insane living habits and practices of civilized man.

It must not be forgotten, however, that as man advances along the scale and the Spiritual Mind begins to unfold, man acquires a something akin to instinct—we call it Intuition—and this leads him back to nature. We can see the influence of this dawning consciousness, in the marked movement back toward natural living and the simple life, which is growing so rapidly the last few years. We are beginning to laugh at the absurd forms, conventions and fashions which have grown up around our civilization and which, unless we get rid of them, will pull down that civilization beneath its growing weight.

The man and woman in whom the Spiritual Mind is unfolding, will become dissatisfied with the artificial life and customs, and will find a strong inclination to return to simpler and more natural principles of living, thinking and acting, and will grow impatient under the restraint and artificial coverings and bandages with which man has bound himself during the ages. He will feel the homing instinct—"after long ages we are coming home." And the Intellect will respond, and seeing the follies it has perpetrated, will endeavour to "let go" and return to nature, doing its own work all the better by reason of having allowed the Instinctive Mind to attend to its own work without meddling.

The whole theory and practice of Hatha Yoga is based upon this idea of return to nature—the belief that the Instinctive Mind of man contains that which will maintain health under normal conditions. And accordingly those who practise its teachings learn first to "let go," and then to live as closely to natural conditions as is possible in this age of artificiality. And this little book has been devoted to pointing out nature's ways and methods, in order that we may return to them. We have not taught a new doctrine, but have merely cried out to you to come with us to the good old way from which we have strayed.

We are not unmindful of the fact that it is much harder for the man and woman of the West to adopt natural methods of living, when all their surroundings impel them the other way, but still each may do a little each day for himself and the race, in this direction, and it is surprising how the old artificial habits will drop from a person—one by one.

In this our concluding chapter, we wish to impress upon you the fact that one may be led by the Spirit in the physical life as well as in the mental. One may implicitly trust the Spirit to guide him in the right way in the matter of everyday living as well as in the more complicated matters of life. If one will trust in the Spirit, he will find that his old appetites will drop away from him—his abnormal tastes will disappear—and he will find a joy and pleasure in the simpler living which will make life seem like a different thing to him.

One should not attempt to divorce his belief in the Spirit leadings from his physical life—for Spirit pervades everything, and manifests in the physical (or rather *through* it) as well as in the highest mental states. One may eat with the Spirit and drink with it, as well as think with it. It will not do to say, "*This* is spiritual, and that is not," for all is spiritual, in the highest sense.

And finally, if one wishes to make the most of his physical life—to have as perfect an instrument as may be for the expression of the Spirit—let him live his life all the way through in that trust and confidence in the spiritual part of his nature. Let him realize that the Spirit within him is a spark from the Divine Flame—a drop from the Ocean of Spirit—a ray from the Central Sun. Let him realize that he is an eternal being—always growing, developing and unfolding; always moving toward the great goal, the exact nature of which man, in his present state, is unable to grasp with his imperfect mental vision. The urge is always onward and upward. We are all a part of that great Life which is manifesting itself in an infinitude of infinitudes of forms and shapes. We are all a part of IT. If we can but grasp the faintest idea of what this means, we will open ourselves up to such an influx of Life and vitality that our bodies will be practically made over and will manifest perfectly. Let each of us form an idea of a Perfect Body, and endeavour to so live that we will grow into its physical form—and we can do this.

We have tried to tell you the laws governing the physical body, that you may conform to them as near as may be—interposing as little friction as possible to the inflow of that great life and energy which is anxious to flow through us. Let us return to nature, dear students, and allow this great life to flow through us freely, and all will be well with us. Let us stop trying to do the whole thing ourselves—let us just LET the thing do its own work for us. It only asks confidence and non-resistance—let us give it a chance.